Psychiatric Aspects of Trauma

Advances in Psychosomatic Medicine

Vol. 16

Series Editor
Thomas N. Wise, Falls Church, Va.

Editors
G. Fava, Bologna; *H. Freyberger*, Hannover;
F. Guggenheim, Little Rock, Ark.; *O.W. Hill*, London;
Z.J. Lipowski, Toronto; *G. Lloyd*, Edinburgh;
J.C. Nemiah, Hanover, N.H.; *A. Reading*, Tampa, Fla.;
P. Reich, Boston, Mass.

Consulting Editors
G.L. Engel, Rochester, N.Y.; *H. Weiner*, Bronx, N.Y.;
L. Levi, Stockholm

Editor Emeritus
Franz Reichsman, Brooklyn, N.Y.

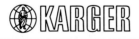

S. Karger · Basel · München · Paris · London · New York · New Delhi · Singapore · Tokyo · Sydney

Psychiatric Aspects of Trauma

Volume Editors
Linda G. Peterson, Worcester, Mass.
Gregory J. O'Shanick, Richmond, Va.

1 figure and 14 tables, 1986

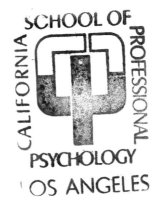

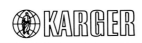

S. Karger · Basel · München · Paris · London · New York · New Delhi · Singapore · Tokyo · Sydney

Advances in Psychosomatic Medicine

National Library of Medicine, Cataloging in Publication
  Psychiatric aspects of trauma/
  volume editors, Linda G. Peterson, Gregory J. O'Shanick.
  – Basel; New York: Karger, 1986. –
  (Advances in psychosomatic medicine; vol. 16)
  Includes bibliographies and index.
  1. Woundies and Injuries – psychology I. Peterson, Linda G. (Linda Gay) II. O Shanick, Gregory J. III. Series
  W1 AD81 v. 16 [WO 700 P976]
  ISBN 3–8055–4219–4

Drug Dosage

The authors and the publisher have exerted every effort to ensure that drug selection and dosage set forth in this text are in accord with current recommendations and practice at the time of publication. However, in view of ongoing research, changes in government regulations, and the constant flow of information relating to drug therapy and drug reactions, the reader is urged to check the package insert for each drug for any change in indications and dosage and for added warnings and precautions. This is particularly important when the recommended agent is a new and/or infrequently employed drug.

Contents

I. Factors Determining Trauma Vulnerability

II. Behavioral Responses to Trauma

III. Trauma Treatment in Practice: The Head Injured Patient

Preface

Disasters, both natural and man-made, affect both masses and individuals. Collective community responses have provided fascinating information for historians, sociologists, and psychiatrists [1, 2]. Nevertheless, psychological trauma has long been a central concept in psychodynamic psychiatry. It is the individual's subjective experience of a traumatic event that is the common focus for the physician. It is surprising, however, that so little attention has been paid to the psychological sequelae of physical trauma. Although stress response syndromes and bereavement receive much attention, the victims of direct physical trauma are infrequently studied [3, 4]. The consultation psychiatrist, however, sees individuals who have been victims of physical trauma either from capricious accidents or brutal, aggressive injuries. It is fitting that two outstanding consultation-liaison psychiatrists, Dr. *O'Shanick* and Dr. *Peterson,* have organized this present volume. It should be carefully read by all who do psychiatric consultations in general hospitals as well as therapists in the psychiatric outpatient arena who treat victims of terrible stresses and survivors grieving for those who perished in such tragedies.

This text would provide an excellent syllabus for a clinical course on Psychosocial Imperatives in Clinical Medicine. Such a course could transcend traditional departmental lines, whether they be surgery, medicine, psychiatry, or pediatrics. It would provide an integrating focus to help the student physician understand the nature of psychosocial response to stress and illness. We should all be grateful to the authors and editors of this text for putting together such important information in one volume. *Thomas N. Wise*

References

1   Lifton, R.J.; Okon, E.: The human meaning of total disaster. The Buffalo Creek
    experience. Psychiatry *39:* 1–18 (1976).
2   Wilkinson, C.B.: Aftermath of a disaster. The collapse of the Hyatt Regency Hotel
    skywalks. Am. J. Psychiat. *140:* 1134–1139 (1983).
3   Horowitz, M.J.: Stress response syndromes (Aranson, New York 1976).
4   Lindemann, E.: Symptomatology and management of acute grief. Am. J. Psychiat.
    101: 141–148 (1944).

Thomas N. Wise, MD, Department of Psychiatry,
The Fairfax Hospital 3300 Gallows Road, Falls Church,
VA 22046 (USA)

Introduction

Trauma is the leading cause of morbidity and mortality up to the age of 34. Psychological and physical sequelae, however, continue to be lifelong problems for many patients necessitating a significant amount of medical care and rehabilitation services. For some, trauma results in chronic disability. Although many trauma victims receive psychiatric care, little systematic attention has been paid to the specific needs of these patients. An increased awareness of post-traumatic stress disorder has emerged since the Viet Nam War, but only recently has this entity been seen as a consequence of nonmilitary trauma. Likewise, many specific types of trauma have been investigated psychiatrically (e.g. burns, amputations, spinal cord injury), but there has been little effort to place these in a more general perspective or to address the multiply-injured patient. In fact, for many years the existence of real psychological sequelae was totally ignored. Post-traumatic neurosis was seen as a primarily litigious condition which could be effectively treated by compensation. This 'fact' dates back to studies of 'railway spine' in the late 1800s which are of questionable validity in this era.

Because of this deficiency in cohesive treatment of the psychiatric aspects of trauma and, further, because of the obvious economic and emotional cost of trauma, this book was conceived. Although one volume cannot adequately address the breadth of the area, the text has been arranged to give differing slices of the field.

The chapters are arranged to give some general consideration of socio-cultural perspective, predisposing causes (i.e. alcohol use), effects of age, and role of families. Following this, major issues in acute management are addressed from a variety of perspectives including major psychiatric issues, and nursing perspectives.

The final section, an in-depth look at head injury, serves as a model of the integrated understanding necessary to all trauma cases if optimal psychological, physiological, and rehabilitative care is to be provided.

We hope this volume will serve as a resource for all physicians and other medical personnel treating trauma victims and sensitize us to the necessity for comprehensive care of these patients.

Linda G. Petersen
Gregory J. O'Shanick

I. Factors Determining Trauma Vulnerability

Adv. psychosom. Med., vol. 16, pp. 1–16 (Karger, Basel 1986)

Trauma: Cross-Cultural Issues

Atwood D. Gaines

Case Western Reserve University and Medical School, Cleveland, Ohio, USA

Introduction

The term trauma has a multiplicity of meanings depending upon the perceived nature of the presenting problem and the frames of reference of the individuals involved. For an event or physical injury to constitute a trauma it must be so interpreted by the participating individuals, the physician, the patient and or the patient's significant others in terms of their respective *weltanschauungen* shared with other culture and or sub-culture mates. Sedimented experiences, too, affect the individual within the framework of his or her culture or these may be unique social and cultural experiences. Psychosocial issues, or even psychosomatic issues, may be profitably viewed as responses of persons which are learned, ·shared and transmitted by particular cultural or subcultural groups composing a society. That is, such responses and interpretations, which constitute patients' behavior relative to medical events, may be seen as psychocultural in nature. They are grounded in common, shared definitions and understandings acquired by individuals as members of cultural groups.

Anthropology, as the social science which treats of the nature of culture and cultural differences may have something to offer clinicians with reference to the understanding of trauma. Cultures are seen in contemporary anthropology as systems of shared understanding embodied and inacted in symbolic systems. These symbolic systems contain central or key symbols [1] which act as models of experience and models for social action [2] in religious or secular contexts. Either of these, depending on the culture, may encompass the medical context

[3, 4]. Cultures, then, may be understood as systems of learned, shared and transmitted meanings, understandings, conceptions and assumptions which are embodied in symbols. Symbols themselves may be persons, places, things, events, gestures, or ideas or anything else that serves as a vehicle for a conception [2].

In the case of trauma, we may observe striking variation across cultures in the events or situations perceived as traumatic. Such differences are grounded in the differing cultures of the individuals participating in the medical encounter. Response to traumatic situations should be seen as meaningful within the semantic system of the individuals concerned; that is, patient and healer alike. In this chapter, several cases are reviewed which point up the wide divergences in definitions of and responses to trauma to be found in various cultures. These cases may also be of use to clinicians whose practice brings them into contact not only with ethnic groups different from their own, but with the folk cultural definitions and theories derived from their own culture which affect patients' behavior.

Other issues to be considered are the potentially hidden meanings and loci of traumatic events. The elucidation of these meanings makes it easier to understand the effect of the trauma on the individual as a part of a larger social system, not merely as an isolated biological unit. In recognizing the significance of the trauma for particular individuals, a distinction can be made between what are generally considered psychosomatic issues and cultural issues properly speaking. That is, psychosomatic issues are not isomorphic with cultural issues and should be distinguished in both practice and theory.

The data presented here derive from a number of sources. Some cases will be drawn from the author's research in France and America. Case material will be used which derives from research on affective states in France [5] and on American psychiatric ideology and practice [6–11]. Also, material will be utilized from the large ethnographic and medical literature containing data relevant to a discussion of the interpretation of responses to trauma.

Trauma

The term 'trauma' conveys several meanings within the medical field. In the original Greek, it meant 'to wound', referring in general to any injury where the skin is broken, but also to injuries where the skin is not actually broken, as in 'head traumas' [12]. In this sense, we refer to traumas of a physical nature.

Freud [13] used the term to apply to events occurring abruptly in which an individual was overwhelmed by stimuli, or by a particularly noxious stimulus such that she/he could neither deal with nor work off the excessive excitations in a normal manner The unexpectedness of a trauma thus increases its potential effect on the individual [14]. In psychoanalytic thought, the impact of the trauma depends upon a person's *Empfänglichkeit,* or predisposition, by which is meant such things as one's state of mind at the time of the event, the social circumstances and situation of the trauma, demands upon the person at the time, and existing psychic conflicts which prevent the subject from integrating the experience into his/her concious personality [12–14].

The psychocultural meaning of and responses to perceived trauma, will be the focus of this discussion. Psychocultural hence will refer to the psychological meaning of an event understood within a cultural, rather than universal, psychological context. This distinction stresses that a person's response is not only individual, but predicated upon meanings, values, conceptions, assumptions and the like which are, in large part, shared with others of the patient's (or healer's) cultural group.

Medicine recognizes, then, two sorts of trauma; those pertaining to physical insults and those insults which are psychically injurious. Both may be seen as psychoculturally injurious, i.e., psychically injurious in terms of a particular cultural meaning system. This classification appears simple, straightforward and commonsensical. However, from an anthropological perspective, it leaves much to be desired.

First, the classification makes the implicit (cultural) assumption that the traumas are located solely within the confines of a physical body, that of the identified patient. Second, the classification defines the problem as uniquely biomedical in nature: that is, existing solely within the physical or biological body and outside of the realm of the mind, or of culture.

The medical anthropological literature provides ample evidence to challenge both points. For example, we know that different ethnic groups respond to comparable injury and pain very differently [15].

Parsons [16] reports differing symptomatology between ethnic groups in matched schizophrenic patient groups. Even classical clinical entities in psychiatry such as depression may be culture-bound illnesses of Western culture [17].

Research also indicates that the Western (i.e. Northern Europe) notion of person found in American Biomedicine is quite distinctive and has implications for definitions of illnesses and treatment strategies [5, 8, 10, 14]. The American concept of person is a cultural conception in which humans are conceived as bounded, physical entities [8, 10, 18, 19]. Further, these entities are seen as distinct from other similar entities and are believed to be the loci of motivation and action [8, 11, 18]. In looking cross-culturally, such a notion of person is quite unusual and distinctive. For example, the Balinese concept of person encompasses spirit siblings [20]. *Shweder and Bourne* [21] did research on the (East) Indian person and found it to be distinct from the American and that levels of education or income did not alter the expressed differences. *Lebra's* [22] work on the Japanese person may be noted here as well as some of the author's work on the contrast between Northern and Southern European person concepts [8, 11] and *Lee's* [23] work on the Greek and Wintu Indian person conceptions. And, we should not fail to mention *Hallowell's* [24] ground-breaking work on the Ojibwa Indian's person conception.

Disease in other societies of the world, including the major tradition of China [3] is, for reasons intimately bound up with person conceptions, frequently located *not* within the 'physical' boundaries of a person so conceived, but rather within networks of social relations [3, 25, 26]. Illness is thus seen as a symptom of disorder in a *social* body, not in an individual, physical body. Hence, therapy is directed toward social groups, not individual 'patients'. In fact, therapy is often conducted in the absence of the identified patient as in Japan, China, Africa and other countries [3, 25].

Group ethnographic and individual clinical examples can be used to demonstrate patterns in the response to trauma and the often overlooked social consequences and involvements of patient's significant others. We will begin by looking at some cultural patterns of response to trauma and then look at specific cases drawn from the author's own research experience and from the anthropological and medical literatures focusing on psychological trauma. However, much of this material can be applied to the more widespread mix of physical and psychological trauma.

Cultural Relativity of Trauma

It is assumed in medical circles that certain events are traumatic in and of themselves. However, it can be easily shown that traumatic events, say of childhood, are not universal. A single ethnographic example will be used to highlight the relativity of trauma. Certain assumptions about trauma which are held in the West may also be questioned by this example, such as assumptions about the negative consequences or sequelea of trauma.

The Iatmul of New Guinea

The Iatmul of New Guinea occupy the Sepik River Valley and practice horticulture along with some hunting and gathering for subsistence. Among this group, studied by the well-known anthropologist *Gregory Bateson* [27], matrilineal descent is practiced. In such a descent system, a woman's husband is an 'in-law', not a relative because he comes from another matrilineal group, which like her own, traces descent only through female lines. In such a system the mother's brother of a given individual (called 'ego' to identify him or her in a kinship diagram) is of cardinal importance because a woman's children belong to her lineage, which is also that of her brothers (but not his children when he marries). The children do not belong to the lineage of their father (who therefore is not a 'father' in the same sense that we intend) as he must come from another, unrelated descent group. In such a society, it is to the mother's brother that the burden of education and the responsibility of the training of his sister's children falls; and it is from him that they shall inherit.

Now, among the Iatmul we find that males can gain prestige by committing murder. Such men, called 'homicides' by *Bateson,* are held in esteem by their peers. So it is that among the Iatmul, the greatest gift that an uncle can give to his nephew, who optimally would be 5 or 6 years of age at the time, is a captive. And, further, the *kindest* of uncles would assist his nephew in the killing of the captive by helping the lad to balance the long spear that serves as the death weapon in such a way that the child is given the credit for the killing. The nephew so gifted by a kind uncle would then be a 'homicide' and a person of considerable social prestige from a very young age.

We might look at an assumption which Westerners might make with regard to the events related above. This is, it would be assumed that these events would have a deleterious affect on the child which would manifest itself in some adult personality problems; a trauma of childhood affecting adult psychosocial functioning. Such theories of the influence on adult psychological organization are held widely, far beyond the confines of psychoanalysis, the field which has thus far best analyzed such noxious influences. Clearly, the Iatmul do not have such a theory. In fact, a great many cultures do not relate events of infancy or childhood to adult psychological organization or social functioning. The concern for 'traumas' among the young is nonsensical in such a context, though Westerners would be hard put not to see murder as traumatic.

This example shows us clearly how different behaviors and attitudes can be in other cultures. Such a radical example moves us off-center and paves the way for understanding more subtle differences in interpretations of behavior. Next, some culturally patterned responses to trauma found in the literature are considered.

Cultural Patterning of Responses to Trauma

Hispanics and Trauma

In certain traditions, such as the Hispanic, it is common for the significant others of an identified patient who has a serious illness to deny the existence of the problem or its severity [28, 29]. Such denial may cause problems for clinicians in that while the patient may not be told of the seriousness of an illness, the significant others, even if told, are likely to deny consciousness of the nature of the sickness or injury. This may lead to serious problems in communication as well as to inappropriate expectations of the instituted medical therapies. The denial of the seriousness by both patient and patient's significant others is thus an example of a culturally patterned response to traumas of a physical or mental nature. The response is a learned, shared and transmitted psychocultural means of dealing with trauma, not an idiosyncratic, psychosocial or even psychosomatic process.

Irish Responses to Death

In traditional Ireland, responses to death can vary greatly depending upon the definition of the nature of the death. Death can be seen as appropriate, or it can be seen as a great tragedy. Critical to the traditional Irish response to the trauma of death is the assessment of the appropriateness of the age of the deceased. If death comes to someone who is considered young, it is a great tragedy. As such, it is a time of great mourning and 'keening' (Irish wailing). However, if an older person dies, one who in the cultural conception has lived a full life (married, farmed, had children and grandchildren), then death and the wake will be occasions not for sorrow or keening, but for joy and laughter. Thus, death *per se* has no constant meaning. Rather, depending on the *social* state of the individual in question, old or young, the response may be sorrowful or joyous [30].

Triste Tout les Temps: A French Grief Response

In contemporary France we find a culturally patterned response to loss which cannot be classified in the American Psychiatric Association's most recent [31] or previous [32, 33] nosologies. Research indicates that a loss of a loved one, or failure in an enterprise in which one has placed great value, can result in very long-term, chronic depressive pictures. In France the term 'triste tout les temps' connotes this condition which could be labeled a 'chronic reactive depression' were there such a label in American psychiatry. The condition seems generally occasioned by some significant loss, as of a child in an accident or even through spontaneous abortion [15]. The condition appears frequently in French literature without any reference to pathology in lay or professional terms [e.g., 34].

This chronic syndrome, with its affective and vegetative disturbances, is neither referred to as depression nor seen as a mental abnormality in France. (The term depression is used in France but it refers to a total collapse of the psyche and presupposes hospitalization.) It is understood as an appropriate response to trauma and is supported by the culture. Case 1 is an example of this.

The support, in terms of acceptance, recognition, lack of stigma and the like, provides for the occurrence of the condition which in turn serves as a model of and for the experience of loss, frustration or disappointment. In the French context, that which would be seen as pathological in America, receives approval by others close to the patient. In this sense the patient and his or her family are part of the same experiential system. In the following, we will consider more closely the possible loci of problems in cases of trauma.

Locating the Trauma

Trauma in the Patient

We may recognize that the trauma experienced can be experienced by either the identified patient or the patient's significant others. The event may or may not be traumatic to the patient depending upon the understanding of the patient of the situation and the seriousness and implications of the particular trauma to the patient. The cases that follow illustrate that trauma may be experienced in ways distinct from that of the attending physician and for reasons not shared with the physician.

Trauma in Significant Others

It should be noted that frequently patient's significant others may be traumatized by particular events occurring to or within the identified patient. The patient should always be seen as part of a social group, the family, or lineage. As such, a disturbance in one component of a system may be expected to generate some disturbance in other parts of the system. Again, the traumatic nature of events derives from the interpretation of events, illnesses or injuries, not from the injuries themselves. There are several levels which may be used to approach the meaning of events, injuries or illnesses to patients and identified others.

On the individual level, one may differentiate a personal set of understandings of the events or injuries perceived as traumatic though these are necessarily based upon shared assumptions and conceptions. Called an explanatory model (EM) by *Kleinman* [3], this set of understandings may be conceived of as a cognitive model which 'explains', for the patient particular aspects of his or her condition. This set of understandings includes etiological hypotheses, the patient's 'theory' about why the event or disease occurred when it did, ideas about the course of the illness, its pathophysiology, i.e. what it's doing in the body or what's happened to the body, about the outcome and appropriate ways of intervening in the illness event.

An understanding of EMs allows clinicians a method for approaching and grasping the cultural dimension of trauma for patients and their significant others. These conceptions allow clinicians to consider cultural questions including those of social/cultural status ('class') when locating, assessing and understanding trauma. The following case material shows the various dimensions, both personal and cultural, of trauma.

Case Material: Responses to Trauma

Case 1: Patterned Response to Trauma of Loss

Research on dysphoric affect in France indicates a patterning of such affect which may be found in other Latin countries, but which is not found in the Northern European Protestant Culture Area. An ethnographic example of this patterning is 'Madame Lorca' who lives in a suburb of Paris. She is the wife of an automobile worker. She was born in a village in Spain, moving with her family to France some 12 years ago. Mme Lorca and her husband have six children. Life is difficult for them; the house is a bit crowded, there is never really enough money and so forth. The children will likely never go off to school or camp like, as she said, '*les vrais gens*' ('the real, true people', i.e., elites) [5].

Mme Lorca herself has experienced a number of traumas in her life. Her life has been sufficiently difficult and her steadfastness in the face of adversity sufficiently strong, that she is referred to as a 'saint' by her many neighbors. Her troubles are well known in her community. Part of the role of the saint is the reinforcing of one's position by the relating to others of current difficulties and the recollections of past misfortunes. In the Mediterranean Culture Area, those who are long suffering and yet virtuous receive a sort of lay canonization. The role of local, or as I have elsewhere termed it, 'visible' sainthood, provides both status and prestige and some power in the tradition [5]. While some of the misfortunes which have befallen Mme Lorca are transient, some are of life-long significance.

Of life-long significance to Mme Lorca were the losses of 3 children through spontaneous abortion over the last 11 years. Mme Lorca speaks not infrequently of these 'babies' who were 'taken from (her) by God'. She bemoans their loss and maintains an object relationship with them. She receives secondary gains from the losses and in fact these losses contribute to her community position as a 'saint', a long suffering, virtuous woman. Her other 6 children provide her with validation for the mother role and reduce to symbolic importance the lost children. Because of the loss of the children, Mme Lorca is described as *triste tout les temps* (always sad), and that she is thus afflicted is reasonable and understandable to her friends, French and Spanish alike.

To assess the nature of her experience of dysphoric affect, clinical instruments were employed. These included the Zung Self-Rating Depression Scale [35], the Research Diagnostic Criteria and the criteria of the Diagnostic and Statistical Manual of the American Psychiatric Association [31]. The instruments clearly indicated the presence of 'severe depression'. However, the research showed that the 'symptoms' of Mme Lorca did not add up to clinical depression. Rather, research demonstrates that there are many people like Mme Lorca in the Mediterranean Culture Area. These visible saints are social cynosures and as such are part and parcel of a cultural system which generates, promotes, patterns and frames the experience of dysphoric affect in a complex which is quite distinct from that of clinical depression [5].

We may see here that trauma is culturally constituted and meaningful and also that there may exist secondary, culturally constituted psychological uses of the traumatic experience. Hence, their occurrence and sequelea are not of necessity solely negative. The management of loss in the case of Mme Lorca is indicative of a culturally patterned, that is, learned, response. It should not be seen as idiosyncratic or 'psychosomatic', the latter in the sense of an unique, individual response.

Case 2: Response of Significant Others to a Psychiatric Problem

A young wife brought her 27-year-old Anglo husband to the emergency room of 'Kahala Kokua Hospital' in Hawaii (1979) for treatment of bizarre behavior including the writing of letters to world leaders in which the husband tells them of his plans for world peace. There was little doubt that the patient was ill, though the patient was unaware that his behavior constituted a problem. However, the most traumatic element of the case was somewhat obscured [8].

The identified patient's wife was very anxious during the examination of the patient by the psychiatric resident on call. Although I noted this anxiety and ascertained its source, the resident did not attend to it, though as he said later, it did 'register in his mind' that she had a problem. His concern was with the identified patient, not with significant others.

The source of the anxiety experienced by the woman derived from the fact that she was uneducated, while her husband was in the process of completing a PhD in chemistry *and* her expectation was that this 'lack' meant that she would be unable to interact successfully with the medical staff. Her greatest fear was that she would be unable to convince ER physicians that her husband was indeed ill. She had little confidence in her social and intellectual skills; she assumed that physicians were above and beyond her intellectual and interactional reach. She saw herself as an outsider and her husband as an insider in the context of interactions with high status care-givers. Her husband's illness thus caused her considerable stress and anxiety for reasons quite different from what one might expect [8]. At one point, the wife asked the resident and I to step outside of the examination room. Once outside, she insisted that we look at letters written by her husband which she had brought along to the hospital. She wanted us to see 'hard' evidence of her husband's illness, as she anticipated that staff would not believe her and would be misled by her husband.

In this case, the patient himself was in fact unstressed, indeed, unaware, that he had a problem. The point here is that the significant other of the patient, the wife, was experiencing stress because of her husband's mental problem (diagnosed as 'manic depression' after a history of fluctuating moods was gathered) which was exacerbated by her fear and expectation that her interpretation of the situation (that her husband was sick) would not be understood or heeded by care-givers whom she thought were 'above' her. Fear of and assumptions about what can be broadly called 'class' differences here engendered a significant portion of the traumatic dimensions of this case. We note that while stressful, the situation was kept from becoming genuinely traumatic for the wife.

Case 3: Response of Significant Others to Chronic Patient's Nonhospitalization

A 41-year-old woman, 'Alice', appeared unescorted in the emergency room of Kahala-Kokua Hospital. She was of Chinese-Hawaiian-Portuguese ancestry but culturally she was 'local', the local amalgamation of various cultural traits which Hawaiian-born people acquire. She was found to have a long history of psychiatric illness, her diagnosis since the age of 16 had been '(chronic) schizophrenia' and she had fairly frequent hospitalizations both at Kahala-Kokua and at the State Mental Hospital. She came to the ER on the orders of her parents who had long accepted that their daughter was 'crazy'. Alice appeared anxious and behaved in a peculiar, child-like manner.

It appeared that she and her family wanted her to be hospitalized but her case did not seem serious enough at first to warrant the utilization of one of only two remaining psychiatric beds at Kahala-Kokua. When asked why she had come to the emergency room, she told the psychiatric resident, the anthropologist and the social worker, all of whom were present, that she had come because she, 'hit my step-father with a plate, (because) he punch me! Hit me. Bruise my back'. This family feud had been precipitated by a relatively innocuous comment which the step-father had made but to which Alice had taken offense and consequently she struck out against him.

During the course of the interview, both the resident and the anthropologist author became convinced that Alice was not schizophrenic; rather, we believed, she was mentally retarded, perhaps having suffered from some brain damage in early childhood. Confirmation was soon forthcoming when Alice's parents called the hospital to see if she had been admitted and the author was able to get a complete history for Alice including an episode of high fever, convulsions and unconsciousness lasting several days.

It was found that none of Alice's relatives, whose identities were learned from Alice, would come to the hospital to take her home. Her parents had likewise refused. It was clear that they wanted her kept at the hospital. After the interview, it was decided by the resident that perhaps Alice could stay in the hospital because she would not be able to get home alone since relatives were unwilling to collect her. Alice, however, did not want to stay in the hospital; she wanted to return home. Since she was not in an acute or dangerous state, the resident was unable to keep her.

When the parents phoned, I was able to talk at length with them. They were very angry and upset that Alice had been let go. They threatened to sue the hospital because we had let a 'crazy' person go. 'What kind doctas you got der, let somebody crazy go?' was one of the mother's often repeated rhetorical questions (spoken in Hawaiian locals' 'Da Kind' talk). The conversation yielded the history of brain damage which did not appear in her medical record. The conversation went as follows [7]:

Anthropologist: . . . Anyway, how long has Alice been like this?
Mother: Since she was 4 years old.
Anthropologist: And what happened to Alice when she was four?
Mother: She got sick. She had a fever and slept for days and vomited and shook. But we lived way out, no doctas, long time ago. But later see docta and he say nothing wrong 'cause she look normal. But there was something wrong, they just didn't understand mental illness then. She never was same after that . . .
Then she went into hospital (state hospital) first time when she was 16.
Anthropologist: I see. Since then, since four, she's had this problem, she's been like this?
Mother: Yea, She crazy.

I suggested to Alice's mother that perhaps her daughter was mentally retarded and not 'crazy'. However, her EM of Alice's condition could make no distinction between the two conditions, both being 'problems in the head'. Her interest was not the new diagnosis, but the *management* of Alice.

Further conversation with Alice's mother showed that her concern and anger was unrelated to a worsening of her state. Rather, the family was trying to get Alice hospitalized because she was becoming too difficult for her increasingly elderly parents to manage. The present attempt at hospitalization was an attempt by the parents, whose understanding of the system was somewhat limited, to find new care-givers for their daughter. This quest was, in part, a conspiracy; it was the reason no one would come to pick up Alice. But more importantly, the situation was very traumatic for the ethnically local parents.

The trauma was experienced in the significant others and was not found in the identified patient. There was the fear that longstanding mental illness would not be sufficiently serious to warrant hospitalization of the patient which would relieve the aging parents from a care-taking task which they felt they could no longer manage. Given their limited understanding of the 'system', they attempted a ruse which did not work. This is an ironic case where *lack* of severity of the psychiatric condition occasioned the traumatic response in the patient's significant others.

Case 4: Parents' Failure to Act Appropriately to Intervene in Child's Serious Medical Condition

The following case of 'neglect' in a traumatic situation was reported by *Jackson* et al. [36]. A young girl became progressively ill. Deterioration due to the presence of ulcerative colitis was noted by a physician who advised the parents on how to proceed. The advice was ignored as the parents instituted a regimen compatible with their religious beliefs (Christian Scientist). Further deterioration finally led the parents to allow biomedical intervention after their retreat into their religious belief system which forbids biomedical intervention. However, the child received attention too late and subsequently died [36].

This case demonstrates how a physical illness can be seen as a symbolic entity. That is, the child's ill health was seen as a test of faith and the rightness of faith's proscription of biomedical intervention. The child is not simply a child, but like all of us, comes from and exists in a particular ideological, cultural context. The responses of her parents are thus framed in terms of their EMs, their perceptions, understandings and assumptions about the nature, course, origin, outcome and appropriate therapy for particular problems. The child's illness may be seen as traumatic to child and parents. But, not only is it a matter of a serious illness in a child, in addition the condition in this society also means for Christian Scientists a confrontation with a powerful medical establishment, equally powerful legal establishments and a test of the family's faith, for they are forced, by their beliefs, to avoid biomedical interventions. Given this ideology in the American context, serious illness entails not only physical difficulties and stress, but as well precipitates social conflict thus exacerbating the already traumatic episode of serious illness.

Case 5: Witchcraft in America – Refusing Medical Intervention

A 40-year-old black woman presented to the emergency department of a large southern university hospital with severe lower abdominal pain [37]. She was kept overnight for observation. Examination revealed lower abdominal tenderness and peritoneal signs. The patient, of a traditional fundamentalist religious background, had an EM of her illness. She believed, and her belief was encouraged and supported by relatives in attendance, that she had been 'hexed', i.e., she had been a victim of witchcraft.

Belief in witchcraft is shared by blacks and whites in the southern United States [38] and cases not uncommonly appear in professional medical contexts. Folk healers, 'root doctors', exist and are well known for their help in these matters. Belief in witchcraft as a cause of illness is also found among certain Mediterranean groups such as Italian-Americans [39]. Due to migrations from the south, these beliefs also exist in other places in the US including Arizona [40] and New York [41].

Since the etiology of the current illness was known to the patient, she had been hexed or 'rooted' ('had a root [evil charm] put on her'), she wished only to leave the hospital. In this patient's EM, the etiology was of utmost significance. Because she believed that she had been hexed, the patient was distraught; she thought she would die unless she could leave the hospital to 'get the root taken off'. She was encouraged in this by her significant others (her sisters). Her sisters said, 'Can't you folks see that she needs help and medical doctors can't treat roots' [37].

Her medical condition, based upon laboratory tests, worsened, indicating that something was seriously wrong and that exploratory surgery was needed. She was advised of the need for staying in the hospital and undergoing the surgery, but the patient and her significant others refused.

During this discussion with the patient, the internist called a psychiatric resident to consult as the discussions of witchcraft had led the internist to believe he was perhaps dealing with a mental problem in addition to an ominous physical problem. The resident was familiar with the anthropological literature on hexing and with fundamentalist religious ideology. His tact was not to deny the validity of the patient's beliefs, which certainly would have resulted in the exit of the patient from the hospital, but rather to work within them to relieve the trauma and to allow for necessary treatment [37].

The patient was told that though she may have been hexed, it would be prudent to stay in the hospital and accept the medical treatment to correct the problem caused by the hex. After treatment for the problem was completed, she could return home and do whatever was necessary to 'get the hex taken off'. This counsel, from an anthropologically sensitive psychiatric resident, produced the patient's compliance with medical advice which, in all likelihood, saved the patient's life as surgery revealed some 140 cm of necrotic, infarcted bowel.

The principal traumatic aspect here is the cause, according to the patient's EM, of the illness episode, not the illness itself. The perception of trauma comes not from an illness in and of itself, but from the symbolic meaning of that illness to the patient and the patient's culture mates. Thus, the locus of the problem is outside the normal, biomedical view and even the understanding of the first attending physician.

Conclusions

The cases presented above show that trauma has different cultural and social meaning depending on the cultural and social (family, class) system in which it is found. As these vary so vary the symbolic/semantic significance of the specific traumatic events or conditions for the people involved. The reality of trauma depends upon complex interpretations which vary in terms of cultural orientation and hence the social responses to, and the recognition of, the loci of the trauma.

The 'reality' of trauma and its very locus depends upon the cultural definitions which the actors have of the events and symptoms, their perceived origins and potential consequences. It is suggested here that trauma should be seen as a psychocultural event occurring within, and indeed created through, the interactions of elements of given social/cultural systems. The elements, assumptions, roles, patterns of defense, the symbolic nature of conditions, etc., may be as significant in the medical picture as the physical presentations of the patient himself/herself.

References

1 Ortner, S.: On key symbols. Am. Anthrop. *75:* 1338–1346 (1974).
2 Geertz, C.: The interpretation of cultures (Basic Books, New York 1973).
3 Kleinman, A.: Patients and healers in the context of culture (University of California Press, Berkeley 1980).
4 Good, B.: The heart of what's the matter: the semantics of illness in Iran. Culture Med. Psychiat. *1977.* 125–158.
5 Gaines, A.; Farmer, P., Jr.: Visible saints: Social cynosure and Dysphoria in the Mediterranean Tradition. Culture Med. Psychiat. (in press).
6 Gaines, A.: Definitions and diagnoses. Culture Med. Psychiat. *3:* 381–418 (1979).
7 Gaines, A.: Knowledge and practice: anthropological ideas and psychiatric practice; in Chrisman, Maretzki, Clinically applied anthropology: anthropologists in health science settings (Reidel, Dordrecht 1982).
8 Gaines, A.: Cultural definitions, behavior and the person in american psychiatry; in Marsella, White, Cultural conceptions of mental health and therapy (Reidel, Dordrecht 1982).
9 Gaines, A.: The twice-born. 'Christian psychiatry' and Christian psychiatrists; in Gaines, Hahn, Physicians of Western Medicine: five cultural studies. Culture Med. Psychiat. Spec. Issue *6:* 305–324 (1982).
10 Gaines, A.: Person and practice among Christian and secular psychiatrists in America. Working Paper No. 1 (Anthropology and Sociology Center of the University of Amsterdam [CANSA], Amsterdam 1983).
11 Gaines, A.: The once- and the twice-born: self and practice among psychiatrists and Christian psychiatrists; in Hahn, Gaines, Physicians of Western medicine: anthropological approaches to theory and practice (Reidel, Dordrecht 1985).

12   La Planche, J.; Pontalis, J.-B.: The language of psycho-analysis (Norton, New York 1973).

13   Freud, S.: Beyond the pleasure principle (London 1950, orig. 1920).

14   Fenichel, O.: The psychoanalytic theory of the neurosis (Routledge & Kegan Paul, London 1953).

15   Zborowski, M.: Cultural components in response to pain; in Logan, Hunt, Health and the human condition (Duxbury Press, North Scituate 1978).

16   Parsons, A.: Belief, magic, and anomie (Free Press, New York 1969).

17   Marsella, A.: Depressive experience and disorder across cultures; in Draguns, Triandis, Handbook of cross-cultural psychology, vol. 6: psychopathology (Allen & Bacon, New Jersey 1980).

18   Geertz, C.: On the nature of anthropological understanding; in Annual editions in anthropology (Dushkin, Guilford 1977).

19   Hahn, R.: A world of internal medicine: portrait of an internist; in Hahn, Gaines, Physicians of Western medicine: anthropological approaches to theory and practice (Reidel, Dordrecht 1985).

20   Conner, L.: The unbounded self: Balinese therapy in theory and practice; in Marsella, White, Cultural conceptions of mental health and therapy (Reidel, Dordrecht 1982).

21   Shweder, R.; Bourne, E.: Does the concept of the person vary cross-culturally? in Marsella, White, Cultural conceptions of mental health and therapy (Reidel, Dordrecht 1982).

22   Lebra, T.: Japanese patterns of behavior (University Press of Hawaii, Honolulu 1976).

23   Lee, D.: Freedom and culture (Prentice-Hall, Englewood Cliffs 1959).

24   Hallowell, A.: The self and its behavioral environment; in Hallowell, Culture and experience (University of Pennsylvania Press, Philadelphia 1955).

25   Turner, V.: The drums of affliction (University of Oxford Press, Oxford 1968).

26   Harwood, A. Rx: spiritist as needed (Wiley, New York 1977).

27   Bateson, G.: Naven (Stanford University Press, Stanford 1956).

28   Kiev, A.: Curanderismo (Free Press, New York 1968).

29   Clark, M.: Health in the Mexican American culture (University of California Press, Berkeley 1959).

30   O'Donnel, J.: The Irish wake. Paper presented at the Celtic Symposium, Department of Anthropology, San Francisco State University (San Francisco 1977).

31   American Psychiatric Association: Diagnostic and statistical manual III (American Psychiatric Association, Washington 1980).

32   American Psychiatric Association: Diagnostic and statistical manual II (American Psychiatric Association, Washington 1968).

33   American Psychiatric Association: Diagnostic and statistical manual I (American Psychiatric Association, Washington 1954).

34   Etcherelli, C.: Elise ou la vraie vie (Folio, Paris 1967).

35   Zung, W.: A self-rating depression scale. Arch. gen. Psychiat. *12:* 63–70 (1965).

36   Jackson, D.L.; Korbin, J.; Younger, S.; Carter, K.J.; Robertson, A.L., Jr.: Fatal outcome in untreated adolescent ulcerative colitis. An unusual case of child neglect. Crit. Care Med. *11:* 832–833 (1983).

37   Lyles, M.; Hillard, J.: Rootwork and the refusal of surgery. Psychosomatics *23:* 1–4 (1982).

38   Hillard, J.; Rockwell, W.: Disesthesia, witchcraft and conversion reaction. J. Am. med. Ass. *240:* 1742–1744 (1978).
39   Foulkes, E.; Freeman, D.M.; Kaslow, F.; Madow, L.: The Italian evil eye. J. operat. Psychiat. *8:* 28–34 (1977).
40   Snow, L.: Folk beliefs and their implications for the care of patients. Ann. intern. Med. *81.* 32–96 (1974).
41   Kimball, C.: A case of pseudocyesis caused by 'roots'. Am. J. Obstet. Gynec. *107:* 801–803 (1970).

Atwood D. Gaines, PhD, MPH, Case Western Reserve University and Medical School, Cleveland, OH 44106 (USA)

Adv. psychosom. Med., vol. 16, pp. 17–30 (Karger, Basel 1986)

Role of Alcohol Use and Abuse in Trauma

Edward L. Reilly, James T. Kelley, Louis A. Faillace

Alcohol Problem Treatment Unit, The University of Texas Medical School at Houston, Tex., USA

Introduction

Throughout history it has been commonly observed that an individual who has suffered some physical or psychological trauma may subsequently develop an increase in his/her drinking. This drinking may in fact become a major and independent problem best viewed as alcoholism. Quite frequently it is virtually impossible to reliably document pre-trauma drinking behavior, since in a retrospective review, both patient and families forget earlier drinking problems. It is often addicts, whether addicted to alcohol or to other drugs, who are involved in accidents, and the increased stress following trauma may exacerbate but not necessarily precipitate addictive drug or alcohol use. Careful initial assessment of the trauma patient is indicated, especially looking for signs and symptoms that suggest chemical abuse and dependence.

Even when the trauma is clearly a suicide attempt, the patient is often drugged or drunk which is, in a large number of instances, an extreme incident within a continuous, chronic pattern of abuse. If the causal or contributory chemical problem is recognized and a confrontation is made, the event can lead to a dual rehabilitation effort. Lack of diagnostic vigor will leave trauma rehabilitation thwarted by increased or at best unchanged chemical disability.

Definition of 'Trauma'

In the broad sense, trauma can be defined as any kind of assault on an individual. This can include the more common physical damage of an auto accident, or the painful emotional upset following an abusive verbal tirade. The traumatic event may be self-imposed, as in a suicide attempt. It may come unprovoked from external sources such as auto accidents, rapes and homicides. The trauma may be the result of alcohol's influence on an interaction between individuals as in fights, homicides, and assaults.

Association of Alcohol Use with Trauma

The association between alcohol use and trauma has been well documented. It has been reported that 64–70% of homicides involve alcohol, and as well as 75% of stabbings, 69% of beatings, and 56% of fights or assaults in homes [1]. If the presence of alcohol in these instances were not associated in any way with the actual increase of violent behavior, then one would expect that the involvement with alcohol would be similar in populations presenting to emergency rooms for reasons other than such trauma or accidents. This is clearly not the case. When breathalizer tests were carried out on emergency room patients, a positive result was observed in 22.3% of the patients involved in home accidents and in only 8.9% of patients presenting with nonaccident emergencies [2]. In this study, the breathalizer test was positive in 56.4% of patients presenting after assaults or fighting. The evidence is fairly strong that alcohol use is prevalent in a large number of patients presenting with various kinds of trauma, and that the alcohol prevalence in such traumatic instances is higher than expected in an average emergency room population.

Physician's Role

In most instances where alcohol abuse problems surface after trauma, initial information about drug and alcohol use was not obtained at the time of the accident. Physicians find themselves examining a person who has been abusing alcohol for from 2 weeks to 2 years post-trauma. The physician's approach to such an individual should be the same as that used in properly approaching an individual whose drinking has no clear antecedent. There must be a confrontation in a nonjudgmental, nonpunitive form. In doing this, the physician must review his or her own attitude about drug and alcohol abuse.

Many consider the diagnosis of alcoholism as a moral judgment which may further alienate the patient. A physician when diagnosing alcoholism or substance abuse should avoid moralizing. A more effective strategy is to inform the patient that he/she has permanently lost the ability to control substance use without outside support. The cause may or may not have been under the patient's control but, once control is lost, this becomes irrelevant as far as treatment is concerned. If the physician is to comfortably and nonjudgmentally inform the patient of a diagnosis of alcoholism, the issue of 'responsibility' and 'punishment' must be faced. This becomes crucial to the patient's general feeling of self-worth and will bear strongly on whether the patient becomes an active partner with the physician in the treatment of alcoholism.

The physician need not get involved in the etiology of the patient's drug abuse as far as treatment plan is concerned. To do so might complicate the issue in relationship to litigation surrounding the traumatic event and impede efforts to stop the behavior. The physician can legitimately tell the patient that it is impossible to determine if the patient's drinking problem occurred secondary to the accident or the inactivity during recovery. By underscoring that the patient's alcohol dependence interferes with recovery from the trauma, sobriety is identified as being in the best interest of the patient so that other aspects of the patient's health will not be further compromised. The physician can point out to the patient that, until the patient is once more chemical-free, the etiology of the dependence is of no importance. Once chemical freedom is solidly achieved (at least 9 months to 1 year of chemical freedom), the causes can be explored in psychotherapy if desired. The critical issue is that the patient's chemical use is harmful to his/her health and retards recovery. This should be explained to the patient as a personal behavior unrelated to any outside agency, and that it is within the control of the patient to change with the help of others. Responsibility is thus removed from the traumatic event and returned to the individual with the problem.

This particular phase cannot be done in a single session but must be repeatedly reinforced. Support of family, friends and, in instances of litigation, the lawyer must be enlisted. These individuals generally are interested in the overall long-term welfare of the patient, but may be concerned that a fleeting or imperfect cure may not be in the best interest of the patient prior to the settling of various compensation claims. All of these well-meaning supporters may add to the chronicity of the condition and contribute biased support in their belief that it is only the result of the previous event. Education needs to be provided that the substance abuse is potentially fatal and detrimental to overall recovery.

Fortunately, the stigma associated with being an 'addict' or a 'drunk' is such that some leverage remains in attempting to alleviate this condition before the patient enters a courtroom. Clear recognition that the prodrome of the state was present before the trauma occurred can be very useful in mobilizing the enablers to accept rapid rehabilitation and recovery rather than attempting to add substance abuse to the list of 'caused ills' of the victim.

If someone is convinced that a series of bad circumstances can cause an otherwise healthy, stable individual to become an alcoholic or an addict, then the foregoing suggestions could be construed as an effort to deprive someone of his/her just recompense. There is, however, no real evidence that individuals 'become' alcoholics as a result of hard times. Such events can and do become the catalyst for an exacerbation of a pre-existing but less evident problem, or, more frequently, provide the opportunity and excuse to use drugs or alcohol to excess. It is crucial for all health care providers to identify the problem rapidly and apply pressure to bring this illness to a halt. The sober individual and the lawyer can litigate and debate at a later date, but the immediate, crucial need is prompt identification and resolution of the abuse.

Some specific types of accidents will be considered separately. The first, because it appears to be the most costly and has the most evident association with alcohol abuse, is auto accident fatalities and injuries.

Traffic Accidents

It appears, at present, that at the very *least* more than half the fatal automobile accidents in the United States are associated with a drinking driver, and in a high percentage of these individuals, there is an alcohol level greater than that of legal intoxication. American society accepts the estimate that half of traffic fatalities are alcohol related. There has been some argument that this 50% figure is quite low, and the American College of Pathologists has made the suggestion that as many as 9 of every 10 fatal traffic accidents involve drunk drivers [3]. The federal figures responsible for the 50% estimate are derived from incidence of fatally injured drivers, but do not necessarily include non-fatal accidents. It has been suggested that if the driver is considered at fault in a fatal accident whether he/she is killed and if single accidents in alcohol-related incidents involving fatalities are included, the relationship of alcohol to traffic deaths may be closer to 90% [3]. This suggests that a blood alcohol level should be done routinely on any individual involved in trauma, especially traffic accidents, rather than only for those who are obviously intoxicated [4, 5]. It is much more useful to know that an individual carrying an alcohol concentration of 150 mg% (0.15%) shows no apparent intoxication than it is to find such a level in a clearly drunk individual as tolerance to such levels is correlated with alcoholism. Similar tolerance at a level of 300 mg% is essentially diagnostic of alcoholism.

Teenagers account for a significant percentage of the fatalities related to alcohol. Ten thousand teenage deaths per year are alcohol related. A number of factors are involved in this high accident rate in teenagers. Although alcohol is a factor, the average blood alcohol level in such teenage fatalities is lower than that found in adults over 25 in such accidents since blood alcohol levels are related to weight not age and conditioning. The other clear suggestion from the high level of mortality related to lower blood alcohol levels in teens is that the teenager is less experienced at driving in general and in driving while drinking, and this is clearly fatal. (It is possible, but not necessarily provable, that the driving patterns of older individuals include greater inter-car distances and less 'bumper tag' giving some greater margin of error.) If one looks at all drivers involved in accidents, at least two-thirds have at least a problem with drinking. Probably half of those receiving their first 'driving while intoxicated' (DWI) citation are not just problem drinkers, but alcoholics needing long-term treatment and rehabilitation to avoid being a serious highway menace.

Driving accidents related to alcohol are not confined to the use of cars. A recent study of snowmobile accidents [6] reported that, of 36 fatalities, drunken driving could actually be excluded in only 6, and for 20 of the 30 drivers from whom blood alcohol levels were available, 17 were in excess of 0.1%.

Swimming Accidents
The role of alcohol in swimming accidents is well documented, but far less recognized and publicized then in traffic accidents [7, 8]. A

number of different factors are involved in this phenomenon. The individual in a swimming accident usually dies alone and in a situation that calls for the involvement of medical rather than legal authorities. The drowning victim is more consistently seen as simply a victim, and there is a tendency to avoid doing anything that might be detrimental or embarrassing to the survivors such as doing a drug and alcohol screen. In spite of the lack of publicity, consistent evidence exists that alcohol plays a role in drowning deaths. This becomes more apparent as the more frequent non-alcohol-related deaths of children are eliminated. The role of alcohol in the drowning deaths of women also appears to be less significant. The figures, if confined to male drowning victims over the age of 15, suggest that at least 35% have blood alcohol levels greater than 0.08% [8]. If an even older population of drowned men is examined, it is observed that in the age range from 30 to 64, 45% of the swimming deaths and 75% of those who fall and slip into the water have blood alcohol levels in excess of 0.15%. The high incidence of drinking to the point where blood alcohol levels suggest intoxication in the adult male has been replicated in a number of studies in Australia, the Scandinavian countries, and England. Such studies in the United States, where alcohol or drug levels are obtained on a routine basis from all victims, are still relatively few, but support the figures from other countries where such routine alcohol and drug determinations have been made on accident victims for a longer period of time and with a larger percentage of the population studied [9, 10].

Swimming fatalities include a number of features that are distinct from auto accidents. Some of the major factors that make swimming accidents potentially more fatal to an unwary drinking individual are the following: (1) unusual amounts of exercises; (2) sudden changes in temperature between outside activity and immersion in the water; (3) a situation where the duration of drinking and the environmental features (particularly temperature) are relatively unusual compared to the drinkers usual drinking environment; (4) a hot, dry environment and consumption of foods with the tendency to provoke increased thirst (such as salted peanuts, potato chips, nachos, etc.); (5) adequate drinking to provoke impaired judgment, thus allowing him/her to decide to go swimming without supervision – in fact, in many instances such people swim with no witnesses who can report difficulty; (6) an activity (swimming) where the individual who develops a problem (cramp, confusion, panic), is not able to simply cease the activity but must make a correct judgment in order to extricate himself/herself from the danger.

Assaultive Behavior

As noted above, various injuries are associated with increased frequency of alcohol use [1, 2, 4, 11, 12]. In general terms, the association between assaultive behavior and drinking can be credited to the decrease in social inhibition, general increase in poor judgment, and increased tendency to express emotion when intoxicated. It should be recognized, however, that the relationship may be more complex than a direct intoxication relationship. Reports demonstrate a high incidence of intoxication both among murderers [13] and among murder victims [14, 15]. Increasing evidence exists that a significant percentage of individuals involved in assaultive behavior were not only drinking heavily but were alcoholics [16, 17]. In one large series, 307 individuals with conviction of assaultive crimes were investigated. Thirty-six percent were problem drinkers, and 70% had previous arrests for alcohol offenses. Only a third of these problem drinkers acknowledged a problem with alcohol, and only 13% had ever voluntarily accepted treatment [12].

The relationship of actual alcoholism to homicidal assaults is strikingly similar to studies demonstrating that 35% of individuals convicted of forcible rape were alcoholics [11]. It is of interest and quite relevant that all of the 'alcoholic' rapists were drinking heavily at the time of the offense leading to conviction in contrast to only 22% of the nonalcoholic rapists. It was also observed that the alcoholic involved in rape is relatively young (26.7 years) in comparison to the average alcoholic in treatment who is more apt to be in the late thirties or early forties.

Trauma Victims

Alcohol intoxication plays a significant role in the assault victim population as well as the population of aggressors. Among homicide victims, as many as 32% were intoxicated at the time of death [15]. In some series, the percentage of intoxication in homicide victims is actually higher than that among suicide victims, who are found to be intoxicated 22% of the time. The association of intoxication and suicide, nonetheless, has been better recognized.

Accidents

As with most other types of trauma, few studies exist where blood alcohol levels are obtained on everyone who presents with a particular type of trauma or injury. However, it is found that among head injuries almost two-thirds of the men and 27% of the women will have alcohol detected in their blood [18]. In burn injuries, positive blood alcohol concentrations have been found varying from 36% [19] to 61% [20]. This high rate of alcohol use associated with injury is not confined to factory or highway; farm machinery fatalities are observed to be associated with positive blood alcohol levels in 50% of those studied, and a number of these individuals so injured had previous revocation of their drivers license because of alcohol abuse which suggest that the problem was not just intoxication but actual alcoholism [21].

Factors Related to Alcohol Use and Recovery

Patients who have had a traumatic injury followed by increased use of alcohol often remark that they did not know what to do with their time. This phenomenon of increased drinking is seen in a variety of settings. It is a problem with executives who do not have clear-cut time expectations or clear-cut goals [22]. It is becoming an increasing problem in the retired elderly, and it is a common problem in the traumatized individual who is not able to return to work, dissatisfied with the situation, and left with no clear-cut expectation as to time of recovery, degree of recovery, or the absolute possibilities of eventually returning to work.

Some of the major factors that contribute to the development of more evident alcohol abuse are: (1) increased discretionary time and boredom; (2) increased enabling 'from family and friends'; (3) negative impact of the 'compensation' issue on prompt recovery; (4) pain, physical limitations, and post-traumatic mood change.

The discretionary time and lack of structure available to the injured individual during recovery can have a significant effect on drinking patterns. This phenomenon is not limited to the individual who has recently suffered a trauma and is seen in the work place where alcoholics are found concentrated in jobs with unclear production goals, freedom to set work hours, and low visibility [23]. The increase in drinking as more time and less structured activities develop is seen in the drinking patterns of alcoholics during vacation. It is particularly noticed in the retirement situation, where drinking, which had formerly been concentrated in the evenings, and weekends, becomes heavier on a daily basis with progressively earlier onset each day.

Concurrently, a decrease in expectations from family members about restrained drinking and the usual insistence on nonintoxicated drinking may evolve. Concern may be focused on the additional problem of excessive use of alcohol, rather than recognizing that the alcoholism, if not confronted, will become a separate, persistent and independent problem that will be detrimental to, and may prevent, timely rehabilitation. Alcoholic and family both have a tendency to attribute the inappropriate behavior to the combination of medications for pain which are taken in addition to the alcohol and thus 'forgive' the alcoholic for inappropriate behavior. In normal social situations, the physician and family both would expect that, if the patient must take medicine which is synergistic with alcohol, then the normal individual should refrain from all alcohol use. This view does not maintain, however, for a person viewed in the 'sick' role, and this lack of restraint becomes detrimental to the recovery of the trauma victim.

Compensation issues have a distinct tendency to prolong the recovery process. This interference in motivation to promptly return to a working, scheduled life exacerbates an individual's tendency to be an alcohol abuser. Whether or not the individual is going to be able to return to his/her old job, efforts to rapidly resolve the uncertainty, lack of scheduling, and lack of social constraints are in the best interests of the post-trauma victim.

The individual experiencing dysphoria not a result of a major affective disorder but secondary to other issues, has a tendency to increase alcohol and drug use in response to unhappiness [24]. Such excessive use is apt to draw the individual further into difficulty. The misuse of alcohol and pain medications makes the individual less able to function. Increasing dissatisfaction with the increasing inadequate function starts a vicious cycle, causing the individual who is prone to drug and alcohol abuse to increase alcohol use with the idea that it will decrease the anxiety related to dysfunction when anxiety is increased in chronic alcohol abuse. The individual who has increased the use of medication or alcohol as an emotional anesthetic finds it difficult to change the circumstance in any way. The person dealing with the common post-trauma theme of pain, alcohol use post-trauma, and drug abuse treatment, must realize treatment can not make a major difference until it is accepted by the patient that chemical abuse is self-destructive and must be eliminated. The need for chemical freedom must become the primary goal in order to achieve other goals, whether those be acceptance of pain, resumption of function, or reestablishment of family and social ties. Many post-trauma victims develop feelings of mourning and depression as described in the chapter by *Brown* [this vol.].

The frequency of the affective disorders leads many individuals to relate the overuse of alcohol or drugs to the affective disturbance rather than the reverse. In fact, if one reviews the drinking behavior of nonalcoholic individuals as they move into a depression, it is found that in most instances a decrease in alcohol use occurs and only a relatively small percentage (7%) will increase alcohol use, much less develop 'alcoholism' [24]. The only major affective disorder that is commonly associated with increasing abuse of alcohol is mania [24, 30]. If, on the other hand, one looks at the response of alcoholics as they develop major affective disturbances, it is found that half or more of these individuals will significantly increase their alcohol use in response to depression, anxiety or psychological tension. Thus, the general tendency to explain increased alcohol abuse and dependency in situations of stress as being a secondary symptom is largely erroneous. Excessive use of alcohol under stress may indicate that the individual, in fact, has a substance abuse problem which is emerging in association with the stress and depression.

The sequence leading to treatment involves, first, the recognition that a problem exists. This recognition generally comes earliest from family who find the behavior intolerable over time. Often, the first complaint is not from family or physician, but from the police when the individual is arrested for public intoxication or driving while intoxicated. It would be far better if excessive use of alcohol was recognized by physicians, but only about 9% of treated alcoholics are referred to treatment by physicians [31]. There does not appear to be any compelling reason to believe that the outreach is any higher for those whose alcoholism becomes the cause of, or more manifest after a traumatic event. If anything, this latter group is better protected and enabled by both family and professionals.

Intervention

When a problem is recognized, treatment team professionals must collaborate with the family in presenting to the patient at a sober moment, their concern and the specific ways that they have seen the chemical use change the patient's behavior. These interventions should include sufficient history with specific examples of times and dates. Such history might include clear evidence of mood change with anger and hostility on specific days of the week. A specific blackout or a specific fall can be cited. The family needs to be educated about the significance of the 'blackout' in which the alcoholic may be talking and functioning in an apparent rational although angry and emotional manner, and the following morning have no memory of the events. If the family does not inform the patient of this, this conspiracy of silence may greatly delay the patient's recognition to the seriousness of the problem. Hopefully the intervention by family and treatment team will lead the patient to an acceptance of treatment.

Treatment

A program for alcoholism generally includes a relatively intensive initial phase followed by a prolonged rehabilitation phase. Attempts to detoxify in 5–10 days are associated with much higher relapse rates than the more prolonged intense efforts over 4 weeks or more. Many programs currently advocate an initial phase of 1 month. While some are totally inpatient or outpatient, mixed programs exist where combined inpatient or intensive outpatient phases (12–20 h/week) run a month or more. Particularly for the post-trauma individual who may still have physical limitations and pain, there is some advantage to an initial inpatient phase in a comprehensive medical center. In such a case, the issues of limitation and pain can be addressed but the focus placed primarily on alcoholism or overuse of drugs. Patients and family require intensive education efforts. Thus, a dedicated alcoholism or substance abuse unit is generally more useful in the initial phase than are attempts to emphasize this focus on a general medical or surgical service. Once the patient is willing to accept that chemical freedom and sobriety is a requirement for maximum rehabilitation, it is easier for him/her to keep the focus on chemical freedom and develop the necessary involvement in support groups such as Alcoholics Anonymous (AA) or Narcotics Anonymous (NA). Frequently, it is necessary to combine some elements of chronic pain programs, including progressive exercise, physical therapy, and biofeedback, in an effort to prevent the patient from being able to 'split' his/her focus by using the somatic complaints as an excuse to avoid looking at the substance abuse issues.

Conclusion

The post-trauma victim is not infrequently found to abuse alcohol and/or medications sometime after the trauma. The frequency of this complication will be reduced if the role of excessive use of drugs and alcohol as part of the initial trauma is more consistently confronted at the time of injury. Recognition that both assailant and victim should have drug and alcohol screens at the time of trauma has increased but is still the exception rather than the rule. Whether or not the trauma was associated with or caused by alcohol abuse, it may provide the setting and the opportunity for the abuser's habit to accelerate to more identifiable proportions. Even if no abuse was present before the trauma, once an abuse situation is recognized, it is critical to confront that issue with the patient and stress the need to focus on this as a primary problem which must be resolved in order to satisfactorily recover.

References

1   Zuska, J.J.: Wounds without change. Bull. Am. Coll. Surg. 66: 7 (1981).
2   Moessner, H.: Accidents as a symptom of alcohol abuse. J. Fam. Pract. 8: 1143–1146 (1979).
3   Alcohol's role in auto deaths stressed. Am. med. News 44 (1984).
4   Maull, K.I.: Alcohol abuse. Its implications in trauma care. Sth. med. J. 8: 1143–1146 (1982).
5   Thompson, C.T.: Alcohol and injury (Injury Prevention Conference). Texas Med. 79: 51–52 (1983).
6   Eriksson, A.; Bjornstig, U.: Fatal snowmobile accidents in northern Sweden. J. Trauma 22: 977–982 (1982).
7   Poyner, B.: How and when drownings happen. Practitioner 222: 515–519 (1979).
8   Plueckhahn, V.D.: Alcohol and drowning. –The Geelong experience, 1957–1980. Med. Sci. Law 21: 2566–2572 (1981).

9 Dietz, P.E.; Baker, S.P.: Drowning epidemiology and prevention. Am. J. publ. Hlth *64:* 303 (1974).

10 Hudson, P.: Alcohol and recreation related deaths. Publ. Safety Sess. (National Safety Congress) *27:* 13 (1976).

11 Rada, R.T.: Alcoholism and forcible rape. Am. J. Psychiat. *132:* 444–446 (1975).

12 Mayfield, D.: Alcoholism, alcohol, intoxication and assaultive behavior. Dis. nerv. Syst. *37:* 288–291 (1976).

13 Goodwin, D.W.: Alcohol in suicide and homicide. Q. Jl. Stud. Alc. *34:* 144–156 (1973).

14 Haberman, P.W.; Baden, M.D.: Alcoholism and violent death. Q. Jl. Stud. Alc. *35:* 221–231 (1974).

15 Abel, E.; Zeidenberg, P.; Regan, S.: Research Institute on Alcoholism, Office of Alcoholism and Substance Abuse, New York Division of Alcoholism and Alcohol Abuse, Uko, J., Rejent, T.A., Erie County Medical Examiner's Office, Buffalo, New York; Division of Surveillance and Epidemiology Studies, Epidemiology Program Office, Violence Epidemiology Branch, Office of the Director, Center for Health Promotion and Education, CDC (1984).

16 Lachman, J.A.; Cravens, J.M.: The murders – before and after. Psychiat. Q. *43:* 1–11 (1969).

17 Carney, F.J.; Tosti, A.; Turchette, A.: An analysis of convicted murderers in Massachusetts: 1943–1966 (Mimeo) (Massachusetts Department of Correction, Boston 1968).

18 Rutherford, W.H.: Diagnosis of alcohol ingestion in mild head injuries. Lancet *i:* 1021 (1977).

19 MacArthur, J.D.; Moore, F.D.: Epidemiology of burns. J. Am. med. Ass. *231:* 259 (1975).

20 Lang, G.E.; Mueller, R.G.: Ethal levels in burn patients. Wisc. med. J. *75:* S5–S6 (1976).

21 LeGarde, J.C.; Hudson, P.: Accidental deaths with farm machinery, North Carolina, 1974. Carolina Forens. Bull. *2:* 1 (1975).

22 Trice, H.M.; Roman, P.M.: Alcoholism and the worker. Alcoholism: progress in research and treatment, vol. 16, pp. 359–382 (Academic Press, New York 1973).

23 Trice, H.M.: Alcoholic employees: a comparison of psychotic neurotic and 'normal' personnel. J. occup. Med. *7:* 94–99 (1965).

24 Wood, D.; Othmer, S.; Reich, T; et al.: Primary and secondary affective disorder: I. Past social history and current episodes on 92 depressed inpatients. Comp. Psychiat. *18:* 201–210 (1977).

25 Akiskal, H.S.; Rosenthal, R.H.; Rosenthal, T.L.; Kashgarian, M.; Khani, M.K.; Puzantian, V.R.: Differentiation of primary affective illness from situational symptomatic, and secondary depressions. Archs. gen. Psychiat. *36:* 635–643 (1979).

26 Guze, S.B.; Woodruff, R.A.; Clayton, P.J.: Preliminary communication-secondary affective disorder: a study of 95 cases. Psychol. Med. *1:* 426–428 (1971).

27 Nelson, J.C.; Charney, D.S.: Primary affective disorder criteria and the endogenous-reaction distinction. Archs. gen. Psychiat. *37:* 787–792 (1980).

28 Weissman, M.M.; Pottenger, M.; Kleber, H.; et al.: Symptom patterns in primary and secondary depression: a comparison of primary depressives with depressed opiate addicts, alcoholics and schizophrenics. Archs. gen. Psychiat. *34:* 854–862 (1977).

29 Mayfield, D.G.; Coleman, L.L.: Alcohol use and affective disorder. Dis. nerv. Syst. *29:* 467–474 (1968).
30 Winokur, G.; Clayton, P.J.; Reich, T.: Manic depressive illness (Mosby, St. Louis 1969).
31 Mendelson, J.H.; Miller, K.D.; Mello, N.K.; Pratt, H.; Schmitz, R.: Hospital treatment of alcoholism: a profile of middle income Americans. Alcoholism clin. exp. Res. *6:* 377–383 (1982).

Edward L. Reilly, MD, Alcohol Problem Treatment Unit, The University of Texas Medical School at Houston, P.O. Box 70708, Houston, TX 77225 (USA)

Adv. psychosom. Med., vol. 16, pp. 31–47 (Karger, Basel 1986)

Trauma in Pediatric Populations

Melanie A. Suhr

Department of Psychiatry, Baylor College of Medicine, Houston, Tex., USA

There are few times in an individual's life span when the impact of trauma is greater than during youth. Accidents represent the leading cause of death between the ages of one and eighteen years and when perinatal complications, congenital anomalies, and pneumonia during the first year of life are excluded, accidents emerge as a significant cause of mortality in infancy as well [1]. Most childhood accidents involve an encounter with a motor vehicle. When not fatal, these and other mishaps often result in major injury requiring hospitalization. The very youth of this cohort underscores the magnitude of productive years lost to death or disability. In many cases, sensitivity to the psychosocial impact of trauma spells the difference between functional impairment far beyond the injury's immediate effects and satisfactory subsequent psychic, social, and future vocational adaptation.

Vulnerability

All pediatricians rapidly become familiar with the occasional child – usually male between the ages of 5 and 10 years – who repeatedly appears in the office or emergency room having sustained an injury. The child 'accident repeater' is defined as any youngster who sustains three or more accidents serious enough to come to medical attention within a year [2]. 'Accident proneness' refers to a more persistent and stable personality characteristic predisposing a child to having accidents [3]. The simplicity of these definitions masks the complexity involved in assessing childhood accident vulnerability.

Personality Traits

Although a specifically accident prone personality constellation has eluded investigators, childhood traits such as extroversion, exploratory behavior, and ready expression of aggression correlate with enhanced liability to accidents [4]. The observation of a higher frequency of mental health contacts among child accident repeaters in comparison with controls has raised the question of whether nonspecific psychosocial maladjustment is not also correlated with increased childhood accident liability [4].

Level of Physical Development

Sensorimotor and neural functioning partially determine vulnerability. Children whose motor skills are accelerated may more frequently find themselves in hazardous circumstances in the pursuit of play activities and the satisfaction of curiosity. Conversely, the child with handicapping conditions which impair mobility, delayed motor maturation, or poor coordination and slow reaction time, may be less able to avoid accidental trauma.

Level of Psychosocial Development

The child's capacity to accurately judge the extent of environmental danger and personal risk relates to the level of his interpersonal and psychic development. In infancy, parents function as the sole guardians of the child's well-being; with advancing maturity, he gradually modulates fantasies of omnipotence and internalizes a sense of danger, using the parents in part as models of self-care [5]. The capacity for self-preservation represents one aspect of emerging autonomous function and certain developmental stages are more clearly vulnerable to accidental injury. In the first 3 years of life, newly found motor capabilities outstrip the toddler's cognitive appreciation of danger and his ability to internalize parental vigilance, rendering him more liable to injury even when effective supervision is present. With age, the child's vulnerability derives from other factors as he leaves the nuclear family for school and peer related activities and is increasingly free of parental supervision. Particularly in adolescence, limit testing and reawakened feelings of omnipotence tend to blunt the sense of danger; the newfound mobility of a driver's license and the introduction to alcohol rise vulnerability to accidental injury during this developmental stage even further.

Level of Cognitive Development

Between the ages of four and seven years, the child's understanding of real cause and effect is poorly formed. Characterized by an incompletely developed ability to differentiate one's own thought processes from events in the external world, the preoperational child's cognition is magical, egocentric, and animistic [6]. Judgments in the face of hazard are often inaccurate and render the preschool child who has already attained some freedom from parental supervision more at risk. With advancing age and maturity, the capacity for concrete reasoning and an increasingly sophisticated appreciation of abstract causality enhance the ability to make appropriate judgments in the face of danger. Intrapsychic issues which emerge either from the pressure of the developmental tasks of adolescence or frank psychopathology may render this cognitive capacity inoperative and produce an increased susceptibility to accidental injury. The same result may obtain in the child whose intellectual capabilities are globally diminished.

Family Functioning

A child's repeated accidents may mask more widespread family difficulties with separation and autonomy [3]. Aside from chronic parental uninvolvement and poor supervision, separation in such families may be accomplished via abrupt ruptures of attachments so as to avoid dealing with the affective issues involved. In other cases, excessive sheltering fails to allow the child sufficient exposure to autonomous functioning and the risks involved. Unless other factors such as peer influence and school educational efforts have compensated for the family's problems, the child receives insufficient supervision, preparation, or instruction in self preservation and emerges more vulnerable to injury.

Exposure to the family stress of illness in another member, parental discord, and other domestic disruption has seemed correlated with a higher susceptibility to injury [3, 7, see also *Leventhal and Midelfort, this vol.*]. Disagreement exists as to whether accidental injuries actually conceal suicidal ideation in vulnerable children [8–10].

Psychic Response to Childhood Injury: General Considerations

The meaning of illness in a child's life depends more on the type and depth of the fantasies it arouses than the nature or seriousness of the condition [11]. The violence, abrupt individual and family impact, and frequent sequelae to traumatic injury, however, are important additional factors in the child's ultimate reactions and adaptation.

As in issues of vulnerability, levels of cognitive and psychological development affect the child's experience of injury. Although most children have a generalized understanding of the hospital's function as that of 'caring for a sick person', their concepts of illness causation and treatment more closely parallel cognitive development as a whole and often fall far short of adult expectations [12]. The preschooler's egocentric thinking leads to self-referential fantasies in which he is guilty and suffering hospitalization as punishment for transgressions. Intrapsychic factors which facilitate this include developmentally appropriate oedipal conflicts accompanied by anxiety and fantasies of retaliation. During this stage, autonomy is tenuous; injury and hospitalization may easily evoke regression. Such a reaction illustrates the vulnerability of newly mastered developmental tasks; at all ages, the most recently acquired skills tend to be the most easily lost under stress [11].

Though theoretical and abstract possibilities are still poorly grasped during the school age era of concrete operational thinking, the child at this level is able to understand more than one dimension of a situation if dealt with in specifics. As a result, he is more appreciative of superficial connections between injury, treatment, pain, and eventual recovery, though he is still prone to regression. In adolescence, the injury and healing processes are increasingly appreciated in terms of internal physiological responses [12]. It is a clinical paradox and a not infrequent source of frustration that increasing cognitive abilities are often opposed by specific psychological reactions congruent with the developmental tasks the adolescent faces. In addition to renewed autonomous strivings that serve identity development, the adolescent must deal with physical maturation and budding sexuality. Body image concerns are heightened. Fears revolving around physical attractiveness and prowess emerge and peer acceptance becomes a prominent regulator of self esteem. The injured adolescent is vulnerable to anxiety, anger, withdrawal, or acting out in the face of bodily damage and enforced dependency in the hospital.

Pre-existing psychopathology, unresolved maturational conflicts, prior experience with illness, and the circumstances surrounding the injury add to the impact of phase specific issues. The developmentally delayed or psychiatrically disturbed child often has relatively inflexible defenses and limited coping skills. Such a child is likely to intensify previous maladaptive responses and resort to regression.

The family's style of child care and general functioning plays a major role in the child's emotional reaction to injury and hospitalization. Some families find such a crisis a rallying point around which they can organize in an effective and mutually supportive manner. Unfortunately, disorganized or rigid family styles are prone to intensification in the face of stress. Parental guilt is a frequent reaction, particularly when the circumstances of injury raise questions about the adequacy of supervision. Some parents find relief in avoidance and denial of potential disability, or in the defensive projection of anger and blame onto medical staff. Disturbances in the child or family need not be seen as pathognomonic of pre-existing pathology, however, as the mobilization of psychological resources required is capable of taxing even the healthiest child and family. It is helpful to consider the entire experience as one which proceeds through certain expectable stages, accompanied by phase specific normal and maladaptive responses.

The Acute Phase

The Emergency Center
The immediate task of this phase is survival and the security of emergency care. Aside from the degree of his maturity, the child's initial psychological reaction to this period is determined by the level of central nervous system involvement, family responses, and severity of injury and pain [13]. Mild forms of trauma requiring only brief emergency care have more limited impact; the child accident repeater may actually deal with minor emergency experiences in a matter of fact manner as his familiarity with the situation increases. For children with more painful multisystem injuries and little prior experience with illness, the emergency room experience is overwhelming. The conscious child easily perceives the crisis response of staff as an overpowering, hostile attack. Emergency centers skilled in handling major trauma are also busy and noisy environments. Careless staff comments and the need for speed impair the child's attempts at preparatory anxiety mastery.

Pain, separation from familiar people, and enforced immobilization feed the child's fears of losing control or suffering mutilation, and augment the impact of environmental stress. Emotional shock, with-drawal and episodic panic herald the presence of a child's acute stress reaction [13], though age and developmental maturity determine the depth of any emotional response; toddlers may be more intolerant of separation from their parents than of pain and stimulation, while teenagers may pathologically deny their injuries in an effort to maintain self-control. Aggression in response to fear may be seen in all age groups, particularly when a clouded sensorium is present. In times of stress, moreover, even older children readily revert to egocentric modes of thinking. It is not uncommon for such a child to believe that all activity revolves around him and all equipment is ultimately destined for use on his body.

Procedures

The experience of anesthesia and the subsequent postoperative period can reinforce fantasies of being overpowered, attacked, or muti-lated. Sensitivity to the level of the child's cognitive and psychic maturity is necessary, for what appears as clearly fantasy in adult eyes is in fact a very real experience for the child.

Pain

The capacity to tolerate pain in childhood is partially determined by previous experiences, the child's grasp of the situation, the quality of his important interpersonal relationships, and the level of his anxiety [11, 14]. The latter is a particularly important issue, evolving from the other three factors. Previous conditioning, fantasies, and the degree to which the child obtains nurturance and parental support determine the child's level of anxiety; pain is poorly tolerated and long remembered when it is reinforced by fear.

Central Nervous System Functioning

Hypoxia or hypovolemia as well as direct head injury may lead to loss of consciousness or subtle changes in the child's perception and orientation and produce agitation and anxiety which augment in-trapsychic reactions. Failing to perceive that his responses are beyond pure 'self-control', parents and medical personnel may be frustrated by the child's failure to respond to verbal reassurance, and risk reacting punitively; this only feeds the child's fears of attack. The experience of an intensive care unit is frequently accompanied by an acute phase of disorientation following the emergence from anesthesia; sensory deprivation, overstimulation, and metabolic disturbances can contribute to delirium as seen in adults [15], but in childhood more subtle central nervous system disturbances may easily be mistaken for provocative, manipulative, acting out behavior.

Family Responses

Clearly the most immediate concern of relatives revolves around the child's chances for survival, but the injured child's family often has added burdens. Frequently, they must maintain the care of other children; other family members may have been injured with the child, and in some instances an important relative has been killed. The family's crisis response is confounded by the presence of multiple emotional demands. Not surprisingly, the relatives of a critically injured child frequently have difficulty assimilating information about his condition and may appear distracted, disinterested, or uncomprehending when it is rendered. Staff may misinterpret these responses as signs of parental neglect and can easily intensify parental guilt surrounding the child's injury if their distortions are transmitted to the family.

Management

When feasible, measures which facilitate the child's mastery of fantasy and fear and restore a sense of direction and competence to the family should be implemented. Preliminary explanation of procedures in simple terms allows the child an opportunity to experience and master anticipatory anxiety and provides him with reality against which he can measure his distortions. The adolescent whose denial is interfering with care may need to be dealt with in a more strategic manner; often complimenting him on his efforts to withstand adversity coupled with encouragement to maintain self-control through cooperation is helpful [13].

A multidisciplinary team approach is invaluable when dealing with families during the crisis [16]. Such a focus streamlines care as it assists in a rapid, accurate assessment of family needs and the timely transmission of information regarding the child's condition. It can also provide much needed structure, particularly when the child has been transported to a trauma center distant from his home and the family is deprived of an extended network of social supports. Attention to parental needs has a beneficial impact on the child's comfort as well, for anxiety in the caregivers is easily translated to the child. The task of such a team at this stage is strictly crisis oriented; more global family issues must await the luxury of time.

The Mid-Phase: Convalescence

Phase-Specific Issues
As the immediate crisis of survival abates, the routine of hospital convalescence begins. Usually, the onset of this phase is heralded by the child's transfer from the intensive care unit to the general ward. The task of this phase is engagement in treatment sufficient to allow healing and eventual discharge. While chronic loss of control, anxiety, intermittent separations, pain, and subsequent procedures may continue, these factors tend to lessen in intensity as new issues emerge to demand the child's and family's adaptation.

Chronic Disruption of Life Routines
Hospitalization separates the child from other relatives and peers and requires parents to divide their attention among the needs of the injured youngster, those of other family members, and employers' demands. At the same time that the hospitalized child is deprived of familiar and comforting family rituals, he is required to tolerate high levels of dependency on strangers in the service of healing. This is especially an issue when orthopedic injuries, burns, or neural axis trauma require prolonged immobilization.

Clearing of Sensorium
With resolution of any acute clouding of consciousness, the child's recall of the circumstances leading up to injury improves unless he suffers a prolonged post traumatic amnesia secondary to head injury. He also becomes more aware of the restrictions imposed by his convalescence. This phase ushers in the acute recognition of changes in his body.

Bereavement
It is during this time that the child is first faced with the impact of others' injuries or deaths. Catastrophic accidents such as housefires or massive motor vehicle accidents often carry with them the threat of such loss [see also article by *Brown*, this vol.].

Common Reactions

Withdrawal, anxiety, regression, and an increased claim for adult attention are common responses during this period. Owing to the young child's incompletely developed appreciation of time, the temporary nature of many necessary restrictions is not fully appreciated; 6 weeks of traction and bedrest seem a lifetime. Once his pain abates, even the most highly functioning child will experience immobilization as a boring and inexplicable intrusion in his life and parents are often sorely pressed to ease his distress.

The acute response to changes in bodily appearance and function depends on the level of the child's self-concept [17]. Prior to age 3, the child's body image is fluid and incompletely formed and bodily changes are dealt with in a more indirect manner. Abrupt loss of functions such as locomotion or sudden changes in family emotional climate precipitated by parental shock, aversion, or grief over the child's losses have more immediate impact than the recognition of bodily damage per se. The older child's body image is more completely formed, however, and his memories of previous wholeness of structure or function evoke responses more similar to adults'. Initially, disfigurement or disability may be denied and avoided. With time and the repeated demands of reality, grief and anger emerge. During this phase, the child may project his rage onto others and may have fantasies or wishes that other children might suffer similar mutilation [18].

Grief reactions in the face of a loved one's death often differ from those seen in adulthood because of the child's immaturity [19, 20]. Younger children may initially seem unmoved by the emotional impact of this loss. The infant whose primary attachment figure is abruptly removed in death, however, shows characteristic protest reactions early. With age, death's finality is better appreciated and grief reactions more closely resemble those of adults [see article by *Brown,* this vol.]. Not uncommonly, the child imagines that he is somehow to blame. The adolescent who loses a peer in the same vehicular accident is particularly vulnerable to this response.

Issues of Clinical Concern

During infancy a prolonged hospitalization may have profound deleterious effects if it is accompanied by an extended separation from major attachment figures. Such a separation need not be the consequence only of direct interruption of physical contact, however. Other family demands, guilt, anger, grief, or aversion to visiting a disfigured child may interfere with parent's emotional availability and effect a psychological separation. The process of intense emotional protest after separation, closely followed by sadness, despair, withdrawal, and emotional detachment, has been vividly described in the literature [21]. Characteristically, the child in the latter phases of such a response seems affectively remote and shows little pleasure in play or feeding activities. With prolonged separation from major attachment figures, self-stimulatory behaviors such as rocking and headbanging ensue and eating disturbances may be so severe as to endanger the child's capacity for physical healing.

Pathological responses in older children frequently derive from the exaggerated expression of common reactions and include prolonged withdrawal, extended dependency beyond that appropriate to the level of impairment and healing, persistent denial or bodily changes, and an inability to relinquish defensive anger and projection. Such responses often mask an underlying depression and are capable of derailing the child from the phase specific tasks of convalescence by interferring with compliance and the gradual resumption of self-care. Children with pre-existing psychopathology or poorly resolved developmental con-flicts are at risk for these maladaptive reactions; for example, the 'hyperactive' child poorly tolerates immobilization, and the child with previously fragile levels of independent functioning may welcome the passivity of convalescence. Poor pain tolerance may signal the presence of adaptation problems.

This period of hospitalization may be complicated by an acute post-traumatic stress disorder [13], a psychopathological entity distinct from the intensification of common responses [article by *Silverman,* this vol.]. Typically, the child experiences episodic intrusive nightmares which engender panic, interfere with sleep, and produce significant debilitation. This disorder may be seen at any age, but is perhaps more clearly recognizable in adolescence where it most closely replicates that described in adults. Detection of the disturbance is more complex in the younger child who has difficulty verbalizing his dreams in a manner that adult staff can understand. The problem may also be less fre-quently suspected in this age group because of the temptation to (mistakenly) explain a young child's anxiety wholly in terms of separa-tion or pain.

Management

Attention to psychosocial issues during this period may often prevent the formation of latter maladaptive patterns capable of short circuiting rehabilitation. Parental 'rooming in' significantly reduces the incidence of emotional protest and withdrawal in infants and young children. When this is not feasible, a consistent member of the nursing staff should be designated as a parent surrogate while frequent family visitation is encouraged. Play activities provide an important avenue of peer contact and allow the child to resume age appropriate tasks while beginning to test out the effects of bodily changes on others. Through play, children may express feelings and act out fantasies which they are only partially capable of verbalizing. When elective procedures are planned, preparatory play activities which enact the anticipated experiences enable the child to sustain and master anxiety in advance. Play tends to oppose overly strong regressive trends as well, particularly when the child is physically able to leave his hospital room for the ward play area. Behavioral contracting and a program of positive reinforcement of compliance can help the hostile child regain his lost sense of self control. Unless he sees such measures in these terms, however, the child will experience behavioral interventions as frustrating, intrusive, and humiliating. Cooperation is enhanced when the process is presented in terms of its competence promoting abilities and the child or adolescent is included as an active participant in selecting the type of reinforcement.

Effective pain management can contribute to overall improvement in the child's adaptation, particularly when the injury is of the type requiring repeated uncomfortable procedures such as wound debridement. When used with medication given in judicious doses and in a timely manner, preparation, distraction techniques, and the presence of familiar attachment figures or adequate surrogates have proven effective in improving the burned child's pain tolerance; hypnosis and self-relaxation techniques may be added for older children and adolescents [14]. These measures easily extend to the management of pain from other injuries as well.

The management of an acute post-traumatic stress disorder is crucial if future chronic phobic anxiety is to be averted. The families of these children, understandably anxious to comfort the child, often encourage renewed efforts at suppression: the child may be urged to keep quiet about his dreams lest they reawaken his panic. This serves the child poorly and does not address the already present underlying breakdown of his defenses. A more therapeutic approach is found in allowing the child to talk about his dreams and fears as he is helped to test their reality [13]. Initially, children may be reluctant to talk about their experiences but the clinician often finds that this material is readily accessible and little prompting is required. The younger child may require the addition of guided play activities which permit him to recreate his perception of the trauma in a concrete fashion. Though tranquilizers may help a particularly troubled child sleep, they must be employed with care so as to avoid reinforcing the notion that renewed suppressive measures are the only pathways to relief.

It is rarely helpful to probe a child's emotional responses to disfigurement and disability early in the convalescent stage. Denial at this point may be adaptive and necessary to maintain hope and the ability to cooperate with care. Psychotherapeutic intervention may be necessary for the child who maintains his denial even in the face of repeated confrontation with the daily reality of his losses. Attention to parental influences in this arena is also essential [18]. If the preexisting parent-child relationship has been conflicted, changes in the child's physique may fan parental rejection and disgust. These feelings are readily transmitted to the child, who is left with few choices; he may internalize his parent's rejection and develop an overt depression, or he may pathologically deny any damage in a desperate bid to regain parental approval. The denying parent also poses problems, as his reaction directly opposes the reality of the child's experience and often leads to confusion and emotional isolation. Family psychotherapeutic interventions may be necessary in these instances.

The convalescent phase makes demands of ward personnel as well, particularly if they become the targets of angry projection. Maintaining emotional neutrality in the face of such a family style becomes difficult; the stress of inflicting pain when procedures are necessary and the need to sustain a positive stance even in the face of gross physical disfigurement take an additional toll on staff morale [22]. Staff cohesion is necessary if these issues are to be creatively mastered; this provides peer support and structural consistency in the face of a particularly hostile family style. It is often helpful to extend multidisciplinary teamwork into this mid-phase in order to comprehensively address all levels of adaptation.

Breaking the news of bereavement is perhaps the most difficult task a family faces during this period [23]. Often relatives imagine that the news will cause the child's physical condition to deteriorate. Usually, however, the child has already noted the deceased's absence among visitors and has in fact come to some tentative conclusions. Delays in informing the child give him yet more opportunity to spin elaborate anxious fantasies and increase the chances of his learning the news from strangers without adequate support. In general, therefore, he should be told as early as possible after his sensorium clears. Despite their anxiety, the parents (or other family relatives in the case of parental death) are best suited to the task. Adequate advance planning should ensure that they have extended, uninterrupted private time with the child afterwards so as to begin to share and mutually support each other in their grief.

The Later Phases: Discharge and Beyond

Phase-Specific Issues

As discharge approaches, the injured child and his family must confront the end of any institutional dependency. Tasks previously performed by ward personnel become the family's responsibility, particularly if they must commit to an extended rehabilitative phase. Positive reinforcement and motivational drives for recovery and functional return, also previously supplied by hospital staff, must now be internalized. Strangers' reactions to lingering visible damages must be confronted. In short, the final phases of adaptation require the child and his family to accommodate to major changes while resuming as near-normal development and family functioning as is possible.

Common Problems

Discrepancies between expectations of immediate return to pre-injury activities and the limits imposed by fatigue, loss of muscle tone, and diminished stamina, may occur in many circumstances. Not uncommonly parents alternate between indulgence and premature insistence on autonomy beyond the level of the child's physical strength. The child himself may unrealistically assume he will be able to rapidly resume prior levels of function; multiple disappointments ensue, making this a trying time for all involved until functional recovery is complete. Additional efforts aimed at closing educational gaps are necessary if the child has not had the opportunity to continue his schooling through a hospital based program. Reentering the world of the classroom also means dealing with other children's aversion or teasing when disfigurement has occurred. If the child is significantly disabled, the family task and role organization undergo major modifications.

Problematic Issues

It is often difficult to distinguish problems which are a function of prolonged hospitalization from those which are a function of the injury per se. The infant reunited with his family after an extended hospitalization may seem 'different': angry, aloof, or persistently detached. Long-term follow-up of older hospitalized children prior to the implementation of rooming-in practices has demonstrated the presence of persistent emotional disruption after discharge [24]. The child whose hospital stay was prolonged has had ample opportunities to perceive the vast amount of gratification and secondary gain associated with the 'sick role', and chronic dependency may result. This clearly interferes with any necessary rehabilitation, as does persistent denial of dysfunction or bodily changes.

Follow-up studies of burned children demonstrate the risks attendant upon disfiguring injury; such children may have serious difficulties reestablishing peer relationships, autonomous functioning, and self-confidence, while their families, particularly mothers, show evidence of chronic guilt, depression, and phenomena suggestive of a chronic post traumatic stress disorder [25–27]. At best, extended effort and special resources are required for the burned child's reintegration into the mainstream of educational experiences with his peers [28].

Nervous system trauma rivals burn injury in terms of long term functional effects. Severe head trauma accompanied by prolonged unconsciousness and post traumatic amnesia is capable of leaving the child with cognitive deficits which may persist over time and adversely affect future learning [see articles by *O'Shanick* and by *Hayden and Hart,* this vol.]. A recent review of this subject suggests that with the exception of disinhibition syndromes similar to those following adult brain injury, clear-cut evidence for psychiatric disturbances specifically generated by brain trauma in childhood is lacking [29] though the degree of cognitive sequelae does correlate with injury severity.

An important complication of major injury in children is the development of a 'vulnerable child syndrome' [30], wherein a child's near brush with death gives rise to major later difficulties. Typically, the child's parents begin an anticipatory grieving process in response to the child's expected death during the original illness; upon his recovery, which may be seen as miraculous, their response is abruptly and incompletely terminated. Such a youngster is seen as snatched from death's very jaws and is treated as though he is forever vulnerable thereafter; the parents actually may believe he is destined to die prematurely. Overprotection and an intense focus on the child's health foster dependency, developmental delay, irritability, and hypochondriasis. Separation anxiety and school phobias may ensue as the child is perceived as unsafe unless under a watchful parental eye. The presence of disfigurement and the chance of peer ridicule may facilitate the emergence of this family disturbance.

Management

Because so much of the long-term adaptation to trauma occurs away from the direct observation of medical personnel, continuity of care after discharge is mandatory if early detection and prompt intervention in problematic responses are to take place. The primary care clinician may spot the development of adaptational failure through close scrutiny of the parent-child interaction on outpatient visits and specific queries related to the child's progress in peer and play activities, schooling, and the quality of self care.

Specialized educational programs are often necessary to allow the child to catch up to his peers and are especially vital to the head injured youngster. Homebound instruction may be appropriate when the child is temporarily immobilized even after discharge but caution and clinical judgement must be exercised. Parental requests for physician approval of such intervention may actually conceal budding problems with separation that are best addressed directly. Outpatient family support groups provide a bridge between the shelter of the hospital and the external world. The process of sharing common concerns and exchanging problem solving methods with others in similar circumstances can promote the family's sense of competence and prevent maladaptive reactions. Concrete positive behavioral reinforcement of the child's cooperative efforts and small successes in rehabilitation is effective in fostering self esteem and keeps the child engaged in this often tedious process. When the above initial measures fail or when a vulnerable child syndrome is firmly established, psychotherapeutic intervention is necessary.

Conclusions

Clearly, childhood trauma has both immediate and far-reaching effects. Intervention after the fact is an essential part of care for the whole child and his family, but should not overshadow primary prevention efforts. Safety education aimed at children must be scaled to the level of phase specific cognitive functioning if it is to have an impact. The use of carseats and other passive environmental restraints can reduce the hazard of childhood injury, as can education about the use of alcohol. Such measures are ineffective, however, if unused; chronically disrupted families whose children may be most at risk are often those most unable to appreciate and make use of public health safety education without added assistance [2, 3]. A high level of clinical awareness of the stresses and risks facing these families is necessary. Collaboration between pediatric and psychiatric clinicians may serve to address these problems, resulting ultimately in care that is truly comprehensive and preventative as well as therapeutic.

References

1   National Safety Council; Department of Statistics. Accident facts, 1982 (National Safety Council, Chicago 1982).
2   Jones, J.G.: The child accident repeater. A review. Clin. Pediat. *19:* 284–288 (1980).
3   Husband, P.: The accident-prone child. Practitioner *211:* 335–344 (1973).
4   Mellinger, G.D.; Manheimer, D.I.: An exposure-coping model of accident liability among children. J. Hlth soc. Behav. *8:* 96–106 (1967).
5   Frankl, L.: Susceptibility to accidents. A developmental study. Br. J. med. Psychol. *38:* 289–297 (1965).
6   Flavell, J.H.: The developmental psychology of Jean Piaget (Van Nostrand, New York 1963).
7   Coddington, R.D.; Troxell, J.R.: The effect of emotional factors on football injury rates. A pilot study. J. hum. Stress *6:* 3–5 (1980).
8   Pfeffer, C.R.: Suicidal behavior of children. A review with implications for research and practice. Am. J. Psychiat. *138:* 154–159 (1981).
9   Shaffer, D.: Suicide in childhood and early adolescence. J. Child Psychol. Psychiat. allied. Disc. *15:* 275–291 (1974).

10   Shaffer, D.; Fisher, P.: The epidemiology of suicide in children and young adolescents. J. Am. Acad. Child Psychiat. *20:* 545–565 (1981).
11   Freud, A.: The role of bodily illness in the mental life of children. Psychoanal. Study Child *7:* 69–81 (1952).
12   Perrin, E.C.; Gerrity, P.S.: There's a demon in your belly. Children's understanding of illness. Pediatrics, Springfield *67:* 841–849 (1981).
13   Ravenscroft, K.: Psychiatric consultation to the child with acute physical trauma. Am. J. Orthopsychiat. *52:* 298–307 (1982).
14   Stoddard, F.J.: Coping with pain. A developmental approach to treatment of burned children. Am. J. Psychiat. *139:* 736–740 (1982).
15   Lipowski, Z.J.: Organic mental disorders. Introduction and review of syndromes; in Kaplan, Freedman, Sadock, Comprehensive textbook of psychiatry; 3rd ed. (Williams & Wilkins, Baltimore 1980).
16   Atkinson, J.H.; Stewart, N.; Gardner, D.: The family meeting in critical care settings. J. Trauma *20:* 43–46 (1980).
17   Stoddard, F.J.: Body image development in the burned child. J. Am. Acad. Child Psychiat. *21:* 502–507 (1982).
18   Watson, E.J.; Johnson, A.M.: The emotional significance of acquired physical disfigurement in children. Am. J. Orthopsychiat. *28:* 85–97 (1958).
19   Furman, R.A.: Death and the young child. Some preliminary considerations. Psychoanal. Study Child *19:* 321–333 (1964).
20   Nagera, H.: Children's reactions to the death of important objects: A developmental approach. Psychoanal. Study Child *25:* 360–400 (1970).
21   Bowlby, J.: Separation. Anxiety and anger (Basic, New York 1973).
22   Quinby, S.; Bernstein, N.R.: Identity problems and the adaptation of nurses to severely burned children. Am. J. Psychiat. *128:* 90–95 (1971).
23   Morse, T.S.: On talking to bereaved burned children. J. Trauma *11:* 894–895 (1971).
24   Prugh, D.G.; Staub, E.M.; Sands, H.H.; Kirschbaum, R.M.; Lenihan, E.A.: A study of the emotional reaction of children and families to hospitalization and illness. Am. J. Orthopsychiat. *23:* 70–106 (1953).
25   Molinaro, J.R.: The social fate of children disfigured by burns. Am. J. Psychiat. *135:* 979–980 (1978).
26   Vigliano, A.; Hart, L.W.; Singer, F.: Psychiatric sequelae of old burns in children and their parents. Am. J. Orthopsychiat. *34:* 753–761 (1964).
27   Wright, L.; Fulwiler, R.: Long range emotional sequelae of burns. Effects on children and their mothers. Pediat. Res. *8:* 931–934 (1974).
28   Chang, F.C.; Herzog, B.: Burn morbidity. A follow-up study of physical and psychological disability. Ann. Surg. *183:* 34–37 (1976).
29   Rutter, M.: Psychological sequelae of brain damage in children. Am. J. Psychiat. *138:* 1533–1544 (1981).
30   Green, M.; Solnit, A.J.: Reactions to the threatened loss of a child: A vulnerable child syndrome. Pediatrics, Springfield *34:* 58–66 (1964).

Melanie A. Suhr, MD, Department of Psychiatry, Baylor College of Medicine, One Baylor Plaza, Houston, TX 77030 (USA)

Adv. psychosom. Med., vol. 16, pp. 48–83 (Karger, Basel 1986)

The Physical Abuse of Children
A Hurt Greater than Pain

Bennett L. Leventhal, H. Berit Midelfort

Child Psychiatry and Center for Developmental Studies, Department of Psychiatry, The University of Chicago, Ill., USA

In the following pages, we describe an important subset of trauma in this country – that which arises from violence within the family and is expressed in the physical abuse of the child by an adult.

As an area of scientific investigation, child abuse is still relatively a riddle, despite a great investment over the past 20 years of energy and funds. In the course of this article, we shall touch on the perennial problems of defining what is meant by 'abuse' and outlining the extent of child maltreatment, as determined by national surveys and expert estimates. After a brief detour to legal history, we proceed to discuss some of the variables which characterize the vulnerable child and family, as well as the effects on the youngster of chronic abuse. Factors which apparently mediate the effects of abuse on later development are discussed and finally practical clinical intervention.

Resources

The literature on child abuse and neglect is, by now, enormous and probably no longer to be mastered (or even read) by any single researcher or clinician. By a variety of means, nonetheless, access to this vast body of information remains possible.

A major database, updated since 1976 annually or semi-annually (depending on the file), is *Child Abuse and Neglect,* produced by the National Center on Child Abuse and Neglect (NCCAN). Containing about 14,000 citations, it is made up of four files – documents, research, programs, and audiovisual materials – and can be accessed by the reference librarians through computer search services at a university or medical center library. Annotated bibliographies on specific aspects of child abuse and neglect are available from the NCCAM Child Abuse Clearinghouse, Aspen Systems, 1600 Research Boulevard, Rockville, Md 20850 (USA). Materials are provided free or at cost. A number of bibliographies on child abuse are already in print, including those of *Polansky* et al. [1], *Kalisch* [2], *Wells* [3], and the National Institute of Justice [4].

The early literature on child abuse tends to have been based on hospital populations (presumably, therefore, more severely injured children) and to have focused upon clinical and case studies. As *Smith* [5, p. 337] has put it recently: 'Stemming from these . . . studies are numerous descriptions of personality traits of abusive parents and situational factors relating to abuse; they have been repeated so frequently that many practitioners speak of them as factual'. Despite ever-constant reminders about the need for adequate sample sizes, control groups, multimodal assessments, and more sophisticated research designs and analyses, it is discouraging to find that the quality of the literature on child abuse has not improved over the past few years.

The leading scientific organization involved in the study of child abuse is the International Society for Prevention of Child Abuse and Neglect (ISPCAN). Its annual membership fee of $50 includes a subscription to *Child Abuse and Neglect*. ISPCAN can be contacted at its headquarters, 1205 Oneida Street, Denver, Co 80220 (USA). Another resource for the clinician, particularly for educational materials dealing with parenting and social action, is the National Committee for Prevention of Child Abuse (332 South Michigan Avenue, Suite 1250, Chicago, Ill 60604, (USA). The NCPCA has chapters throughout the country.

Research summaries and statistical analyses of high quality are the hallmarks of the Children's Division (recently renamed 'The American Association for Protecting Children') of the American Human Association, 9725 East Hampden Avenue, Denver, Col 80231 (USA). For some time now, the AHA has tabulated reports of incidents of abuse nationwide and has disseminated the findings in an annual report and overview of developing trends. There is one other excellent recent review of the literature by *Friedrich and Einbender* [6].

Definition

Implicit in the Child Abuse Prevention and Treatment Act of 1974 is that the effects on the child, not the abusive characteristics of the act itself, should be the determining factor. The American Bar Association's Juvenile Justice Standards Project [7] took the matter further by suggesting that general harm to the child should be evident in some physical disfigurement, impairment of bodily function or other serious injury, while emotional damage must be shown, for example, by the child's 'severe anxiety'. It is no easy matter, however, to substantiate 'mental injury', a concept which, since 1977, federal law has required to appear in the child abuse statutes. Subtle emotional abuse is not readily documented, unlike the more dramatic cases of emotional damage for instance, failure-to-thrive.

Research definitions of child abuse have usually followed one of two tacks – either they presume abuse because of the very fact that an incident has been reported to a state agency or else they insist on an excessively narrow, explicitly behavioral criterion. Both approaches ultimately invite a lack of comparability across studies. The former definition is probably simply not valid. The latter, while quite verifiable, is impractical. It tends to be seen as too lengthy and cumbersome for widespread use.

What are some of the elements essential to devising a research definition?

Inclusion or exclusion of 'neglect' as part of abuse is a difficult issue as is the involvement of a particular causal theory in the definition. The reader is referred to the following discussions of these two areas: *Wolock and Horowitz* [8]; *Fontana* [9]; *Gil* [10]; *Silver* et al. [11]; *Polansky* et al. [1]; *Giovannoni and Becerra* [12]; *Steele and Pollock* [13]; *Aber and Zigler* [14], and *Valentine* et al. [15].

Incidence

In light of the problems in defining child abuse and the inconsistencies in the use of terms, the estimates of incidence are themselves inconsistent. In the early 1960s, *DeFrancis* [16] found 662 cases of child abuse in newpaper reports in 48 States and the District of

Columbia. Based on data collected in 1965 by the National Opinion Research Center (NORC) from over 1,500 respondents, *Gil* [10] estimated the national annual incidence of abuse at between 2.5 and 4 million cases. *Light* [17], who re-analyzed *Gil's* data and applied the same rate to information from the 1970 census, offered a somewhat lower estimate of physical abuse: between 200,000 and 500,000 incidents annually. The issue of the precision of these figures is demonstrated by the fact that the NORC survey had found just 45 people who said they personally knew families involved in incidents of child abuse that, within the preceding 12 months, had resulted in physical injury.

Data from child protective agencies nationwide from calendar year 1983 [18] shows over one million reports of maltreatment. This was a 8% increase over 1982; the number of children involved increased 15%. The National Committee for Prevention of Child Abuse [19] estimated that in 1984 there had been over one and a quarter million reports of child abuse (including sexual abuse). For the 31 States in which data were available for 1983–1984 as well as 1984–1985, the number of reports showed an increase of over 19%! The 'true' incidence rates for child abuse and neglect are far from having been determined. There is general agreement, nevertheless, that, if we are subject to error, it is probably that of significant under-reporting.

Types of Abuse

Common types of injuries inflicted upon abused children include bruises, abrasions, lacerations, burns and fractures [10], drowning, poisoning, and visceral [20]. Minor physical abuse is approximately ten times more frequent than either major physical injury or burns. One hospital-based study of over 300 cases of abuse to children aged less than 1 year [21] found the typical features of the 'the battered child syndrome' (subdural hematoma, long-bone fractures, and soft-tissue swelling) to be present in about a fifth of the sample. *Friedrich and Einbender* [6] have, also, summarized this area as well.

Based on a sample of approximately 400,000, the American Association for Protecting Children [18] found the following breakdown of types of maltreatment:

Major physical injury	3.2%
Other physical injury	23.7%
Sexual maltreatment	8.5%
Emotional maltreatment	10.1%
Deprivation of necessities (food, shelter, etc.)	58.4%
Other (including abandonment)	8.3%

Because of some overlap, the figures total over 100%.

Reece and Grodin [20] provide guidelines for distinguishing between highly suspicious injuries and those which seem genuine accidents, prompted neither by intentional nor – insofar as one can make this judgement – unconscious hostility to the child.

Demographic Characteristics

Early demographic data on child abuse was derived from hospital-based research [21, 22]. A nationwide survey was done before the changes in child abuse reporting laws [10]. The best current survey is the National Study of the Incidence and Severity of Child Abuse and Neglect, sponsored by the National Center on Child Abuse and Neglect [23b]. The annual reports of the American Human Association (AHA), provide reports from child protective workers with a broader spectrum of abuse than hospital data [23a].

Age

Studies based on emergency room admissions show that at least two-thirds of children seen are less than 6 years of age [21, 22]. According to some, as many as 60% of abused children are less than 2 years of age [24–26]. *Gil's* [10] data as well as those from the AHA [23a], suggest a bimodal age distribution for the physically abused – young children, on the one hand, and adolescents on the other. Three-quarters of the children in *Gil's* nationwide sample were over 2 years of age and one-fifth were adolescents. The AHA reported 40% of the abused and neglected children in their sample were less than 6 years old [23a]. *Gelles and Straus* [27], similarly, reported two peaks in parental violence: the

3–4 year olds, the youngest in their sample, and 15–17 year olds, the oldest. Very young children, who are apparently more susceptible to severe injury, may be overrepresented in the statistics. Of those severely or fatally injured, *Gil* [10], for example, found 65% to be under age three.

Gender

Most studies report no significant difference in the proportion of males to females subjected to child abuse [21, 23a, b, 24, 26]. Gill [10], however, reported boys to outnumber girls in every age group up to 12 years, after which the number of abused girls nearly doubled that of boys. From adolescence onward, it is possible that the physical abuse of girls is associated with sexual abuse. There is some controversy about this in the literature [28]. Moreover, the power differentials shift in adolescence; teenage boys are less likely to submit to physical abuse without putting up a struggle that could exact its toll from the would-be abuser [29].

Ethnic Differences

Most studies have found that the abuse rate among non-white families exceeds that which would be expected on the basis of their representation in the US population [23]. These findings may reflect confounding factors such as poorer socioeconomic conditions among non-whites, ethnically divergent childrearing practices [30], discriminatory attitudes among law enforcement and other professional personnel, and differences in reporting practices.

Family Size

The family child-to-parent ratio is generally higher for the boy or girl at risk for abuse. In a recent year, some 43% of the reported cases of abused children came from single-parent (usually female) households – this, in the face of data from the 1980 Census in which such households account for only 14% of the total nationally [23]. Abused children tend also to be a part of a larger than average family [10]. The issue of family size is, of course, often related to poverty and ethnicity. As a factor in child abuse, one must also consider the implications for good child care of having too few adult caretakers or too little time for any one child [5].

Abuse of Others in the Family

In some sense, child abuse may be a means or style of parenting which is generalized to other children in the family. *Gil* [10] reported abuse of more than one of the children to have occurred in nearly 30% of the families in his study. In their sample of families, *Herrenkohl and Herrenkohl* [31] found that 50% had more than one target of abuse. The question of whether the 'identified patient' is somehow unique – either as a 'scapegoat' or because he or she is somehow inviting victimization – bears on how one conceptualizes child abuse. Transactional models [32] seem most plausible. One should not preclude the possibility that a certain child may be more likely, for any of a number of reasons, to be the principal target of and participant in a cycle of violence.

Recurrence of Abuse (Recidivism)

Between one-third and one-half of the abused children in sampled populations are said not to be new cases; they had been abused before [21, 22, 24, 25, 31, 33]. *Herrenkohl and Herrenkohl* [31], who studied the records of 286 verified child-abusing families, found that two-thirds had a second recorded incident of abuse and over half had 2–5 additional incidents. A significant association was also noted between young age and recurrent abuse. This may be one area of child abuse where the figures may be suspiciously high, rather than underestimates. The subsequent injuries, at any rate, are usually less severe than the original one [34] with re-injury rates ranging between 20 and 30%, depending on the study.

Socioeconomic Status

The original claim of equal distribution of abuse across all socioeconomic categories has, for many, capitulated to the demonstration that the largest proportion of abusing families is relatively poor [35]. It may be, however, that the maltreatment associated most clearly with poverty is the neglect of children, not their abuse [8]. The relationship of social class to abuse is still a matter of controversy [36]. *Lenington* [37], who compared census information with data from the surveys of *Gil* [10] and the statistics of AHA [23a], concluded that the rates of child abuse are highest for young male children from poor families. Family income continues to be cited in recent studies [38, 39] as, at the very least, an important factor in establishing a setting conducive to parental violence.

Social Context of Abuse

As noted above, most reviews of the available evidence have concluded that child maltreatment is concentrated among socially, economically, and psychologically 'at-risk' families. Indeed, according to *Elmer and Gregg* [40], the environment of childrearing has more of a destructive influence on a child's development than the specific acts of mistreatment themselves. Two different kinds of social environments are of importance – one outside the family, the other within it.

The Neighborhood
The socially and psychologically damaging climate in which maltreatment occurs would make adequate child development difficult in any case [42]. The mutual interaction between families and their social surroundings can undermine family functioning [43]. Abusing families, in fact, exist in an already compromised social setting. According to a national representative survey of violence against children [44], the incidence of such violence is directly and significantly related to 21 variables indicating social-situational distress and a history of social deprivation. These results confirm the findings of *Garbarino and Sherman* [45], who examined data on rates of maternal child abuse/maltreatment for 58 counties in New York. The degree of socioeconomic stress on mothers without adequate support systems, he found, accounted for 36% of the variance in child abuse rates; more general economic conditions affecting the family accounted for another 16%.

In analyzing the social context of child abuse, some investigators have invoked the concept of a 'neighborhood risk' as mediating between particular family variables and the broader social context. *Garbarino and Sherman* [46] matched two neighborhoods, one high-risk, the other low-risk, on the basis of information from 'expert' informants. Samples of families were interviewed in each neighborhood (22 in the high-risk, 24 in the low-risk area) to determine the balance of stresses and supports, with special emphasis on sources of help, social networks, residents' evaluation of the neighborhood, and the use of formal family support systems. A consistent pattern emerged whereby the high-risk neighborhood could be characterized as relatively socially impoverished. In each of eight aspects of the neighborhood (e.g. its public image, its 'quality of life', and its neighboring and informal supports), interviewee comments were seen by a 'blind' evaluation to favor the low-risk area. The mean 'stress' scores for families – based on the Holmes-Rahe Adjustment Scale [47] – were also significantly different: They were in the 'moderate crisis' range for those in the high-risk neighborhood and on the lower end of the 'mild crisis' range for those in the low-risk counterpart ($p < 0.05$). In coping with these stressors, mothers in the low-risk areas were more likely to include professionals among the people they called upon for assistance.

The difference in family life as a function of the neighborhood were striking. In over four-fifths of the families in low-risks areas, for example, children returned home from school to a *parent;* this was true only of a quarter of the cases in the high-risk neighborhood ($p < 0.05$). Parents in the low-risk areas were also more likely to use the neighborhood for appropriate playmates for their children. Mothers in the low-risk neighborhood, also, rated their area as a better place to live, childcare as more available to them, and their children as easier to raise. What *Garbarino and Sherman's* [46] study does not tease out is a specific 'neighborhood effect' on the high-risk families. Would any given family be more at risk in one neighborhood than in another? High-risk families, after all, are most likely to live in high-risk neighborhoods, both because of their personal histories and because of the political and economic forces that shape residential patterns and encourage people to form clusters [48, 49].

Parent-Child Interaction

As opposed to more static variables, the parent-child interaction is a dynamic, evolving variable in the development of abuse. *Dietrich* et al. [50] observed 53 mother-infant dyads during a feeding session. The children were drawn from five diagnostic groups – nonaccidental trauma combined with failure-to-thrive, nonaccidental trauma combined with iron deficiency anemia, nonaccidental trauma only, neglect only, and normal control subjects. The relationships in dyads in which the child had been subjected to maltreatment were found to differ qualitatively from those in the other groups. The element of mutual engagement best accounted for the differences. This factor indexes the extent to which the mother and infant are sensitive to, responsive to, and involved with one another [51]. Abusing mothers are less active and less stimulating than are nonabusing mothers.

Wasserman et al. [52] videotaped the free play of 12 abusing and 12 control mother-infant pairs, matched for infant age, sex, race, and socioeconomic status. The child abusers were more likely to ignore their infants and less likely to initiative play with them, move about, and use verbal means to teach infants about aspects of their environment. In comparison to nonabusing mothers, they were also less positive in their interactions, they showed more negative behaviors and fewer indications of positive affect.

A recent study illustrates the paradoxical behavior of 'abusing' mothers in reference to their children. *Fontana and Robison* [53] analyzed 10–12 min of videotaped interaction between 8 mother-child pairs, where the mother had been reported for having seriously abused or neglected her children. There was a control group of similar size, four of whom were in the same hospital, but not in the temporary shelter and with no known history of child abuse. The children ranged in age from 9 to 18 months. The abusive mothers were found to be engaged in many activities directed towards the child – they were, in fact, intrusive and almost relentless – yet they focused *on* the child only relatively little. They seemed intent on prompting a response from the child and spent about twice the time the others did in initiating activities. Previously abusive mothers were more likely than the others, as well, to interrupt or distract the child from what he or she was already doing. They were either simply insensitive to affective cues from the child or unwilling to attend to the signals.

The security of a child's attachment is another important relationship variable relevant to the etiology of child abuse and neglect. There is at least indirect evidence for this. A longitudinal study by *Blehar* et al. [54] of a normal sample of 26 infants found that the infants later identified as anxiously attached had been more unresponsive and negative early on than were securely attached infants. Their mothers, similarly, had been more likely to be impassive or abrupt. In their reactions, moreover, the anxiously attached infants also had not differentiated much between their own mothers and an unfamiliar figure. This 'superficiality' would provide less pleasure to (if not actually anger) a primary caretaker. One cannot help but wonder if, for that very reason, some of these 'unrewarding' children sooner or later get abused. We know that children *already* abused are unrewarding and unresponsive in just this way.

In a structured play situation, *Gaensbauer and Sands* [55], for example, observed 48 mistreated (abused and/or neglected) infants and a cohort of 100 nonabused children from 6 to 36 months of age. Compared to normal infants, they found, the abused and neglected children demonstrated: (1) social and affective withdrawal which might be experienced as a rebuff; (2) lack of the pleasure so important to the development of caretaker-infant bonding; (3) inconsistency and unpredictability; (4) shallowness or fickleness; (5) ambivalence/ambiguity in affective expression, and (6) negative affective communications. *George and Main* [56] were even more precise in contrasting the social interaction of 10 abused preschoolers, ages 1–3 years, with that of 10 matched control children from stressed but nonabusing families. The abused children and infants were found to be more aggressive towards their peers and their caretakers, both physically and verbally. There were also differences in approach and avoidance. In most instances, there was clear evidence that a friendly invitation from either a caregiver or another child put the abused children into an intense approach-avoidance conflict.

Abused children approached the teachers only half as often as did the control children and were much less responsive to a friendly move from either caregivers or peers. Only 2 of the 10 abused infants responded to overtures from caregivers by turning to look at them; all ten of the control children did. When they approach, the victims of abuse were more likely to do so indirectly, i.e. by side-stepping or back-stepping or coming from the caregiver's side or from behind her. Abused infants also avoided caregivers about three times more frequently than did controls.

The study of *Blehar* et al. [54] demonstrates that later disturbances in affective communications can be traced to dysynchronous and unsatisfying interactions with caretakers beginning very early in the child's life. Whether the original dysynchrony results from constitutional factors in the child, from inadequacies in the parent(s) or from both, the consequences are by no means transient. Personal characteristics, once established, take on a life of their own; they affect the child's entire environment, including his or her caretakers. Rather than being a merely passive recipient, the infant/child should, therefore, be viewed as an active participant in his or her destiny. This applies, as well, to the child subjected to abuse and neglect.

Legal History

Because child abuse and neglect are criminal acts with legal ramifications, they presuppose a system of laws with an established balance between the rights and perogatives of the child, the parents, and the State. In fact, the legal status of children has been evolving for thousands of years [57]. American law, has closely paralleled the developments within British law. By the second half of the 19th century in this country, the state had taken an interest in safeguarding children against being severely beaten or cruelly or inhumanely treated [57]. In 1874, the case of Mary Ellen Wilson, an 8-year-old girl who had been abused and neglected by step-parents, gained enormous press coverage and consequently mobilized the public spirit. Less than a year following the disclosures of the details of Mary Ellen Wilsons's life, the Society of the Prevention of Cruelty to Children was founded. By 1877, the American Humane Association had been incorporated. By the turn of the century, it comprised 150 anticruelty or humane societies nationally dealing with both child and animal protection.

Since World War II, medicine has become increasingly concerned about certain of the phenomenon of the intentional abuse of children by parents. Since the publication of 'The Battered Child Syndrome' by *Kempe* et al. [58] and the ensuing media coverage, the issue of child abuse has remained a matter of great public concern [59]. By 1967, all the States had passed child abuse reporting laws. Seven years later, the Federal Child Abuse Prevention and Treatment Act became law. From 1974 onward, this legislation has provided for substantial and direct financial support to the States in the form of grants for innovative programs, the training of personnel, the founding and maintenance of centers, and the provision to communities of teams of consultants.

Today, the concept of 'presumptive parental rights' prevails. It is assumed that the parent's and child's rights are the same and that a parent wants to act in the child's best interests. Only when the facts of a case dramatically indicate otherwise is this presumption abandoned. The child has the right of *not* being totally denied an education, of *not* being neglected to the point that his or her life or health is imminently threatened, and of *not* being punished to the extent of endangering physical well-being. These 'negative legal rights' come into play only when parental behavior drops below some acceptable standard.

The standards (e.g. the level of parental support to which a child is entitled) have not been spelled out. Equally problematic is the child's lack of access to society's purview from birth until beginning school; identification of need, therefore, has tended to rest by default with the parents. Except in cases of possible loss of liberty (e.g. incarceration) or juvenile court cases, furthermore, the child often has no right to independent representation. The law continues to evolve. More and more, it is centering on the child as an individual with needs independent of and different from those of the parents and as a person entitled to societal protection.

Developmental Effects/Outcome

Neurological Sequelae

Retrospective studies of samples of mentally retarded and samples of abused children suggest a decided association between physical maltreatment and neurological problems. *Buchanan and Oliver* [60], for example, who surveyed the records of 140 children in two hospitals for the mentally retarded, estimated that 3–11% of the children had been rendered retarded as a result of abuse. According to *Caffey* [61], violently shaking infants is related to chronic subdural hematomas which, he speculated, leads to retardation. *Martin's* [62] report of a 3-year follow-up study of 42 abused children tentatively supports *Caffey's* hypothesis: Among the children who were functionally retarded, a history of skull fracture or subdural hematoma was four times more common than in the remainder of abused children, who had normal IQs. Eight of the 13 children with major physical injury (i.e. skull fracture with subdural hematoma) scored in the retarded range on standardized tests.

In a follow-up study of another sample of children, 4.5 years after the instance of physical abuse, *Martin* et al. [63] discovered that about half had positive neurological findings. These ranged from evidence of mild gross and/or fine motor incoordination, hyperactivity, dyspraxia, and perceptual or sensory distortions to significant functional handicaps in the form of paresis, impaired cranial nerve function, and focal signs. Fifteen of the 31 who had neurological dysfunction also had a history of skull fracture or subdural hematoma. Of the remaining 37 in the sample with no such history, 16 still manifested neurologic dysfunction. In interpreting these data one must remain cautious. Neurological problems is abused children may either have preceded the abuse and/or been caused by it [64]. As will be shown in the following section, abused children come into the world with more than their share of biological disadvantage, including birth defects and a tendency towards early illness.

Other Medical Problems

Besides suffering the direct sequelae of adult mistreatment, the abused/neglected child is also at increased risk for a whole variety of other medical problems. Apparently, the abused child begins life at a disadvantage which is later compounded by ongoing care of inferior quality and consistency. In comparison study of abused children to their nonabused siblings, the mistreated children had an increased incidence of congenital abnormality, as measured by rates of admission to a special care nursery, and much higher rates of illness during the first year of life, including both severe illness and recurrent minor health problems [65]. Abused children may also be more likely to be premature. *Herrenkohl and Herrenkohl* [31] found a statistically significant tough small correlation ($r = .12$; $p = .05$) between target status and premature birth when comparing those targeted for abuse with their nonabused siblings.

It may be that prematurity, as such, is not the determining factor. In a recent study in which the possibly confounding element of poverty was held constant in both groups, *Hergenroeder* et al. [66] carefully matched 40 children, 33 of whom were known to have been physically abused, with 40 'controls'. The study subjects, in the main, were black, male, and less than twelve months of age when the diagnosis was made of abuse, neglect or failure-to-thrive. Although there was more prematurity in the study group than among the controls, the differences were not statistically significant. What differentiated among the children was the study group's (1) greater incidence of low birth weight relative to expected weight, and (2) their higher rates both of admission to the neonatal intensive care unit and of having to remain in the hospital after their mothers had been discharged. The latter two characteristics are, no doubt, clinical consequences of the first.

Hergenroeder suggested that underweight full-term infants are at once less attractive to vulnerable parents, irritating in their monotonous and high-pitched cries, difficult to soothe and nurture, and relatively unresponsive to caretakers. However, the relationship to later physical abuse even of low birthweight is still an open question. The case-control study of *Leventhal* et al. [67] found neither variable to be significantly related to child maltreatment. The authors did not deny that low birthweight and/or prematurity might make for a difficult early adjustment to parenting – but the problems, they argued, may not be long-lasting. At any rate, *Leventhal* et al. [67] cited several other studies that also show that it remains to be proven that these factors figure importantly in an outcome of abuse.

McCabe [68] has argued that another factor in child abuse may be a misleading age-level indicator, based on cranial/facial proportion, which prompts the parent to have unrealistic expectations of the child. Such expectations not being met might prove one of the triggers for violent rage against the youngster. In measurements made both on actual children and on photographs in two independent samples, physically abused 3 to 6-year-old children were found to have cranial/facial proportions that made them look somewhat older than their chronological age. It remains to be seen whether very young abused children also show the 'misleading' and salient age-level indicator evinced by those of preschool age and older. *McCabe's* [68] hypothesis seems more convincing, at any rate, for potentiating the risk to older children, not infants.

Ongoing lapses in child care (e.g. lack of immunizations, inadequate hygiene, and erratic treatment for illness) are seven times more frequent among abused children than among victims of accidental trauma [69]. In the same vein, there is evidence that abused children are more at risk for ingesting any of a variety of poisonous substances [70]. *Martin* [71] described several physical correlatives of abuse which have yet to be substantiated by the research. He noted that anemia is more common in abused children, even in infancy, most likely due to an inadequate supply of iron-containing foods.

Martin's observations and those of others suggest that mistreated children are also at increased risk for hearing deficits. The hearing problems may be directly related to the effects on injuries to the head or may be secondary to chronic, untreated, otitis media [72]. Even in infancy and early childhood, hearing problems could interfere with language and cognitive development. As importantly, the diminished communicative capacity would be likely to invite further abuse at the hands of an impatient, frustrated, and angry parent.

Intellectual and Cognitive Status

It seems the consensus that the IQ scores of physically abused children are lowered [73] and that their language is delayed [74]. Since abuse and neglect often coexist, the research findings for abuse alone are not definitive, however. Most studies did not screen their abused samples for evidence of neglect, whose detrimental effects on all areas of development, including intelligence, are well known. Clinical research in the 1960s and early 1970s had suggested that about a quarter to a half of abused children were classifiable as mentally retarded [40]. Over two-fifths of the small sample studied by *Morse* et al. [33] were found to be mentally retarded three years following hospitalization for illnesses and injuries judged to be sequelae of abuse or neglect. One-third of 42 abused children in another 3-year follow-up study were functionally retarded, with a developmental quotient or IQ of less than 80 [62].

Some studies have included comparison groups in examining the effects of child abuse on intelligence. Typically, the subjects have been infants and toddlers. *Gregg and Elmer* [33] compared 30 infants, less than 13 months of age, suspected of having been abused with 83 children of same age and low SES categories thought to have suffered accidental injuries. About two-fifths of the abused as compared to about one-fifth of the accidentally-injured children were assessed as retarded. If a subsample of 17 children from each of the above groups is any indication [75], both groups had had similarly adverse health status at birth, but at the time of the trauma the abused children had weighed less, had more overall health problems, and showed more negative and variable moods. The children did not differ in distractibility, activity level, mental language, or motor development.

At 8 years follow-up, two comparison groups were added to the study to control for the different hospitalization experiences the abused children and the accident victims had had. In visual-motor coordination and academic achievement, the 'high certainty' abused subgroup (n = 12) did worse at follow-up than the few 'low certainty' abused children (n = 5). The 'high certainty' subgroup also had significantly poorer teacher ratings than did the 'low certainty' abused and the matched accident comparison groups. There were no significant differences between the main groups in a variety of language measures. Close to three-quarters of *all* the children, other than those in the control group, had one or more language problems. *Elmer's* [75] study may reflect the effects of family and neighborhood violence and the underlying problems of severe poverty which affected all the families studied, even the 'non-abused'. Functionally, these life conditions create a shared subculture of chronic parental distraction which, for many children, constitutes a kind of ongoing neglect which cripples language development [76].

In another infant study, *Appelbaum* [77) compared 30 abused children in the beginning of their second year of life with 30 nonabused infants, matched for age, sex, race, and socioeconomic status. The abused infants scored significantly lower on Bayley Scale cognitive and motor measures. Their scores were also significantly lower on three of the four factors on the Revised Denver Developmental Screening Test, personal-social, language, and gross motor. *Appelbaum's* findings were partially confirmed by *Koski and Ingram* [78], but *Dietrich* et al. [79], who compared 14 abused infants with 14 matched, nonabused controls, found that mean scores on the Bayley Scales for *both* groups were within the normal range. Six of the abused versus only two of the control group, however, were more than one standard deviation below the mean on both scales. The group mean scores on the Mental Scale also differed significantly in favor of the controls. With regard to older children, in two different evaluations with the McCarthy Scales, 6 months apart, *Fitch* et al. [80] compared a small sample (n=9) of abused children 2½–8 years of age with a matched control group (n=5). The two groups differed significantly in the predicted direction. The results of a later study using the McCarthy Scales were generally confirmatory [81].

In the study of *Barahal* et al. [82] of abused children between the ages of 6 and 8, the abused children (n=7) had group test IQs (Slosson Intelligence Scale for Children) well within the normal range ($\bar{X} = 102$), but the control group (n=16) scored significantly higher ($\bar{X} = 112$). As the sample of abused children in this study was without neurological impairment and did not typically come from economically disadvantaged families, these findings are of special interest. In a recent and well-controlled study [83] of equal numbers of abused children, neglected children, and those with no such history (14 in each group, from 3 to 6 years of age), there were significant differences between the controls and each of the maltreated groups on the Stanford-Binet Intelligence Scale, the Peabody Picture Vocabulary Test, and the Merrill-Palmer

Scale. The scores of the abused and neglected children, however, were rather similar.

With regards to school success, the impression is the same. In a large retrospective, follow-up study, *Kent* [84] compared 219 child nonaccidental trauma victims with 159 neglected children and 185 low-income controls. All were under the jurisdiction of the Juvenile Court in Los Angeles at the time of follow-up. The age ranges of the children were not stated. Case-workers who carried a maximum of three such cases and were blind to the child's group placement completed a questionnaire for each child. A little over half of the abused group and about four-fifth of the neglect group were assessed to be doing below average or were failing in their schoolwork. This was true of only a little over a quarter of the controls. Whatever the vulnerability to criticism of many of the studies of the effects of abuse on intellectual development, one cannot dismiss the general finding of impaired intellectual function. The findings are particularly strong for infants, if somewhat less clear with regard to abused preschoolers and older children.

Language Development

The early literature on child abuse suggested an association with delays in language development. All of *Martin's* research with different samples of abused children reports lags in language development. Using the Revised Yale Development Schedules (RYDS) and the WISC to study 42 abused children, *Martin* [62] discovered 16 of them to have language scores 15 or more points below their Full Scale IQs. Using the RYDS to evaluate another small sample, *Martin and Beezley* [85] reported overall normal scores, but mean language developmental quotients at the bottom of the low normal range. Although *Blager and Martin* [74] found the scores of a small sample of abused children to be average or better on a variety of standardized tests, they reported that the syntactical quality of the children's speech was still an average of 11 months below expectations based on chronological age. Neglect may be the factor of importance in creating deficits in language as suggested by *Elmer's* [75] prospective follow-up of 17 abused and 17 nonabused, accident victims matched for age, sex, race, and SES. At follow-up 8 years after the trauma, with two comparison groups having been added to the study, 70% of all the children in the groups other than the controls had one or more problems with language.

Personality Behavioral Characteristics

Studies on the behavioral and emotional characteristics of abused children suffer from significant research design deficits.

Clinical Studies. Abused children have been described as aggressive and full of hatred [53]; uncontrollable, negativistic, and subject to severe temper tantrums [86]; lacking in impulse control [87] and withdrawn and inhibited [88]. Those who have observed (assaulted) children in their homes or elsewhere describe them variously as depressed, passive, and inhibited, as 'dependent' and anxious, and also as angry and aggressive. The children fail to participate in play and show little or no enjoyment. Expression of feeling is often so low-key that it is easy to overlook; or else ambiguous and contrary [40, 55]. Crying may be prolonged and unresponsive to comforting; anger is easily aroused, intense and not readily resolved [89].

For *Bowlby* [89], anxious attachment is a key explanatory principle for what at times seems an utterly inconsistent presentation (inhibited yet impulsive, affectively low-keyed but unconsolable, at once passive and aggressive). *Blumberg* [28] seemed to have been aiming at the same analysis, but he emphasized the centrality of childhood depression resulting from various forms of deprivation. The continuity and pervasiveness of aggression in the lives and personalities of the abused child are illustrated by the study of *Lewis* et al. [90] who compared, among other things, the neuropsychiatric histories of extremely violent versus less violent incarcerated boys. At a proportion of roughly 4 : 1, significantly greater numbers in the more violent group had been physically abused by adult relatives and family 'friends' and had witnessed extreme violence directed at others. The degree of these boys' violence was correlated with their own history of physical abuse. The more violent group, moreover, demonstrated psychotic symptoms and had a greater number of both major and minor neurological abnormalities. Presumably, some were the result of physical maltreatment.

The clinical lore about abused children is only partially supported by more rigorous search, as the following discussion indicates.

Empathy. Data on empathic capacities are inconsistent. In their study of a small sample of abused children 5–10 years old matched with controls, *Straker and Jacobson* [91] found the maltreated group to be significantly less empathic, as well as more maladjusted. *Barahal* et al.

[82] also described their group of abused children as relatively handicapped, in comparison to nonabused youngsters, in affective and cognitive role taking, empathy, and social sensitivity. In an imaginative piece of research on moral and social judgement, *Smetana* et al. [92] compared abused, neglected, and nonmaltreated preschoolers who were matched carefully on the variables of intelligence and social class. Among the few differences elicited by the study, the varying attitudes and conception among the two maltreated groups were the most striking. The abused children, in fact, seemed more sensitive to psychological distress in others. The neglected children, as might be expected, were more responsive to the moral wrong of the unfair distribution of resources.

Aggression. It seems unarguable that physical brutality against children begets aggressiveness in the victims. *Green* [93] studied 60 abused, 30 neglected, and 30 control children, ages 5–12 and found the abused children to be more aggressive than the neglected children, who tended more towards passivity and apathy. *Reidy* [94] found that abused children (mean age 6.5 years) expressed significantly more fantasy aggression and used aggressive behavior with much greater frequency in free play and in TAT stories than did comparable groups of neglected children or controls. On the Behavior Problem Checklist, however, both the abused *and* the neglected children were judged by their teachers to be more aggressive than the controls. *Hoffman-Plotkin and Twentyman* [83] confirmed this finding, but still emphasized that, relative to children who had been neglected, the abused children were significantly more aggressive, more socially interactive, and more likely to be the subject of teacher discipline.

Body Image. Abused adolescents are reported to have a significantly impaired body image [95] and have been distinguished from nonabused adolescents on the basis of projective tests, e.g. the house-tree-person [96]. One cannot avoid noting that some projective tests, particularly drawings are of problematic validity and that a broad concept like 'body image' cannot, in any case, be encompassed by a single measure [97].

View of the Family. Using the Family Relations Test, two different investigations on small samples [81, 97], found abused children to think of themselves as unliked and unappreciated by their parents. What is interesting is how much affection for the abusing parents is nonetheless retained by abused children. In interviews with abused (n = 14) and nonabused (n = 10) boys, ages 8–12, who were residents in a group home [99], most of the abused children reported feeling excessively punished by their abusive parent(s), but nonetheless loved and cared for. *Bowlby's* [89] notion of anxious attachment seems to be confirmed by these findings.

Other Effects. Important and deleterious long-term psychological effects of physical abuse are, however, suggested by a number of retrospective studies that show histories of physical abuse to be overrepresented among delinquents [100–102], abusive and violent parents [100, 103], and among men who batter their wives [104]. There has been a rash of recent case reports, as well, of children and adults with multiple personality who present with a history of severe abuse [105–107]. Corroboration and a deeper understanding of these findings await rigorous and well-controlled follow-up studies of samples of abused children.

Oates [108] traced 39 children, averaging 9 years of age; 24 boys and 15 girls, who had been hospitalized, on the average, 5½ years previously. In all but 4 cases, the youngsters had been admitted at the time with evidence of varying degrees of physical abuse. Each child in the study group was very carefully matched with a control from the same school. Even after the presumably abuse-free interval, the abused group reported themselves to have fewer friends than the control children. They seemed more inhibited and shy (Children's Personality Questionnaire) and less esteeming of themselves (Piers-Harris Scale). Teachers, who were blind to the purpose of the study and did not know of the children's histories, still rated the abused group's classroom behavior as more disturbed and disturbing. Mothers' perceptions were quite similar. While the abused group was no means severely handicapped in all areas – it did show clear differences from the controls.

Mediating Variables

Over the past two decades, researchers have tried to identify variables which mediate or influence the psychological effects of abuse. In this connection, *Kinard* [109] has distinguished between the sociodemographic characteristics of the victim and the characteristics and history of the abuse itself. We shall briefly review some of both kinds of mediating factors.

Age. The younger the child, the more likely that abuse will result in aggression turned toward others. *Martin and Beezley* [85], for example, found that parental punitiveness was associated with aggressive behavior in children at all age levels but that the direction of the child's aggression varied. With age, extrapunitive responses decreased and intropunitive responses increased [110]. The finding may even extend to the content of fantasy. According to *Rolston* [88], fantasy aggression occurred more frequently in children who had been abused before age 3 than in children abused at later ages.

Gender. The role of the abused child's gender on later outcome is probably governed by his or her absorption of socially determined and differential expectations of the response to parental aggression. Based on a review of the literature, *Feshbach* [111] concluded that boys are more likely to respond to severe punishment by exhibiting overt aggression, whereas girls tend to react with more inhibited, possibly more passive behavior. Girls, at any rate, are apparently more likely than boys to show conflict and anxiety about feeling or showing their aggression.

Family Size. A family-size effect has been reported only by *Goode* [112], who found that larger families tend to use physical punishment more often than do small families. Indirect reasoning would lead one also to expect more incidents of excessive and uncontrolled punishment in the larger families.

SES. Middle-class parents are thought, by middle-class social scientists, to prefer the use of psychological punishment. Lower SES parents are said to be more likely than their middle-class counterparts to use physical punishment in rearing their children; they are also supposedly more tolerant of aggressive behavior in their children. *Smith* [5] has briefly summarized some of the literature on the issue of social class-related forms and standards of discipline and punishment. It is by no means clear that child abuse is more prevalent among the poor simply because of their traditional preferences for handling children. Stress and isolation from extra-familiar supports [36, 113], among other factors, may be more important elements in making poverty and social class so apparently crucial a mediating factor in the later outcome of abuse.

Attachment to Parents. The necessary research in this area waits to be done. Although many speculations about the effects of who abuses, mother, father, or other could be made, there is no available data to support any theory.

Characteristics of the Abuse. The severity and particular type of abuse experienced by the child are important to consider in understanding later outcome. Physically disfiguring scars or neurological deficits can be expected to carry with them a relatively higher risk of accompanying and enduring psychological stress [114]. The frequency and the degree of the predictability of the abuse are likely also to be important for the longer-term effects on personality. According to *Rohner* [115], persistent and severe rejection results in flat affect and apathy.

Although perhaps difficult to characterize for the purposes of research, there is a form of purely emotional abuse which, experienced as parental rejection, must have extreme consequences for personality development. Emotionally abused children have been found by *Rohner* [115], for example, to be hostile, aggressive, or passive-aggressive and to consider themselves worthless and unlovable. *Martin and Beezley* [85] found that children subjected to both physical and verbal abuse showed more psychiatric symptoms than children who had been less harshly punished. The child's response in the course of his or her development, one could argue, is not specific to the form which the mistreatment has taken, but just to the fact of the ongoing abuse. There is evidence, however, that some responses to certain kinds of maltreatment are more typical than others. Mention has already been made several times to differences between abused and neglected children.

Children may react to neglect with apathy, passivity, withdrawal, and flat affect or with hostility, anger, and aggression [1]. The effects of sexual abuse are likely to vary with the circumstances under which it occurs [116]. As the child grows older and realizes the inappropriate and exploitative nature of an intrafamilial sexual relationship, she or he may feel used and worthless and may become unable to trust others. The sexually abused younger child may exhibit regressive and infantile behavior or withdraw into fantasy worlds. Adolescents may also exhibit increased aggresive behavior [117].

We have only touched upon forms of adult cruelty other than physical abuse. There are, no doubt, similarities in the dynamics of child maltreatment that apply to all its different manifestations. More importantly, it is quite likely that where one form occurs, others do – either in combination or over time. It is hard to think of each in pure culture.

Interventions

A multitude of interventions have been suggested for abused children and their families. Indeed, the literature in the field regularly recommends that multiple interventions be applied to each case of child abuse. These suggestions appear in the face of relatively limited data supporting the special efficacy of any particular intervention or interventions in the treatment of child abuse.

Although there are different types and possibly even different causes or disposing factors for child abuse, there is a framework for intervention which are common to most, if not all, treatment programs:

(1) Protection – acute intervention to protect the child from additional insult or injury.

(2) Acute medical/surgical care – immediate institution of measures to deal with injuries and other acute medical problems.

(3) Reporting – reporting child abuse or neglect to the appropriate agency, when required by law.

(4) Environmental assessment – rapid assessment of the child's and family's environment.

(5) Diagnostic evaluation – comprehensive evaluation of the child and family.

(6) Treatment program – long term, comprehensive intervention.

(7) Evaluation – assessment of the efficacy of the intervention.

Protection is the most immediate need of the abused child. Preventing further physical injury to the child is essential, of course, but protecting the child from further neglect and minimizing further psychological trauma are also critical. Since it is often difficult, under conditions of acute distress, to assess the safety of a child for the immediate future, 'protective custody' may be the only option available. While removal of the child solves the acute problem, it itself increases the longer-term risks attendent upon separation from family and other social supports. Rules pertaining to protective custody vary from jurisdiction to jurisdiction, but the principle of emergently removing the child from a hostile environment must be followed. Only after the child is safe can the rest of the evaluation proceed.

Acute medical care should include a careful and complete physical examination of the child. While it is often difficult under such trying circumstances, the examination should attend to both the acute and the chronic problems of the child and should be carefully and explicitly documented. Since it is quite possible that the results of examination will be a part of legal proceeding, they should be carefully and legibly recorded. When appropriate, photographs of lesions should be obtained, as well as pathological specimens. In the case of alleged sexual abuse, an appropriate genital examination should be conducted, paying particular attention to possible perineal injuries as well as to physical evidence of the abuse (e.g. loose pubic hairs, fingernail scrapings, VD screen, and vaginal swabs for sperm, phosphatase and ABO typing). Acute treatment of all medical problems is essential even in the face of resistance from parents.

Reporting child abuse to a governmental agency is required in every state, although the rules and form of the reporting process vary with the jurisdiction. Nationwide, the principle is generally the same. In most cases, the law requires reporting of 'suspected' abuse; the report leads to an investigation by the governmental agency. Failure to report child abuse in most states is a violation of law and may be grounds for civil and/or criminal penalties. Clinicians must be aware of the requirements and formats for reporting abuse.

Environmental assessment is necessary before determining the best setting to provide for the abused child. There are usually a variety of alternatives, e.g. a brief pediatric hospitalization, a foster home, and a shelter. Since every setting has its own virtues and limitations, it behooves the clinician to be familiar with the unique characteristics of each prior to making a disposition.

Most often, the abused or neglected child is initially evaluated or detected in the pediatric emergency room. As a result, the initial step is often immediate hospitalization for the purpose of protecting the child. While expeditious, such a move may not be optimal. Many factors and persons protective of the child may already exist in his or her natural environment. Before removing the child from familiar surroundings, one should consider whether such a recommendation might, in fact, constitute aggravation of the situation. In cases of sexual abuse, for example, it has been suggested that the child stay in the home and the allegedly offending adult(s) be made to leave. If this is not possible, one should still consider other temporary arrangements which would leave a child near his or her friends, siblings, and school. Placement with grandparents, family friends or other responsible adults could not only assure the child's safety under conditions which disrupt his or her life relatively little, but also assure continued participation in the evaluation process.

Removing an abused child from the home is a serious decision and a controversial one. Some experienced clinicians [20] seem to believe that separation is often necessary. Others are more reluctant:

> '... Despite the speculative nature of the prevalent conclusions about the developmental sequelae of child abuse, professional warnings support a practice of separating children from their natural homes in the interest of their and society's protection. They focus professional concern and public wrath on "the untreated families" ... and may justify punitive action to save us from their children. The lack of knowledge, or, perhaps more accurately, the inadequate understanding of the state of knowledge promoted by the anxiety which child abuse stimulates in all of us, is translated to recommendations for intervention, many of which are heavy-handed, unspecific, and insensitive, and some of which are downright harmful' [118].

In the event that home-based protective care is not possible, other community options must be carefully scrutinized. Not all foster placements, shelters and pediatric wards are havens for the frithtened and abused child. Some degree of personal acquaintance with these facilities on the clinician's part is necessary before making the placement recommendation. A careful history, furthermore, can help fit the placement to the strengths and weaknesses of the particular child. In any case, it is often wisest to keep the child close to community supports such as other family members, school, friends, and church. With the disruption softened, treatment is facilitated.

After providing acute medical care and establishing a protective environment for the child, a careful and complete *diagnostic evaluation* of the child and family is essential. Such an evaluation is the basis for establishing and monitoring a treatment program. Because child abuse is so repugnant, it all too easily can become the focus of the clinician's view of the child. As a result, other crucial characteristics and problems of the child may be overlooked. A diagnostic evaluation allows for time and attention to be turned to the 'whole' child so that a more balanced picture can be gained.

Many abused children are 'at-risk' for other pathology, as noted previously. The evaluation should therefore include all the elements of a complete examination, including detailed history of the presenting problem, complete review of the child's developmental and past history, complete family history, review of systems and physical examination, psychiatric examination of the child, examination of the family members, psychological testing, and other specialized examinations and consultations as indicated.

Within the limits of the situation, the diagnostic evaluation should develop a complete determination of the physical and mental functioning of the abused child and his or her family. When diagnostic criteria for specific disorders are met, these should be noted. The multi-axial DSM-III diagnostic system is particularly useful because it directs attention not only to the medical diagnoses but also the 'highest level of adaptive functioning' (axis V) and to 'psychosocial stressors' (axis IV).

Integrating the findings of the diagnostic evaluation into a *treatment program* is perhaps the most difficult step in working with the abused child and his or her family. Abusiveness appears to be a recalcitrant feature of relationships within certain families. There are relatively few studies to guide us in choosing interventions which best help the family to change. In her excellent review of behavioral interventions with abused children, *Smith* [119] has noted that 'child abuse is *not* a unitary phenomenon'. Thus, a single or uniquely 'appropriate' treatment is not likely to exist or be forthcoming. In a review of eleven treatment projects, *Cohn* [120] found that only about 40% of over 1700 patients were felt to have shown a decreased potential for abuse, despite multiple interventions at the hands of several professional and lay support staff. Furthermore, when specific outcomes related to target behaviors were assessed, the proportion of successful problem resolution dropped to 28%.

In the face of ever-growing numbers and the absence of a proven intervention strategy, the treatment literature is replete with suggestions for every and all forms of treatment. Therapies of all sorts, whether alone or in combination with other treatment, have claimed at least short-term efficacy for parents, families, and abused children. A good rule to follow is that the primary determinants of the treatment protocol are to be found in the diagnostic process. In the initial stages of the treatment process, one should identify the elements necessary to prevent further abuse and insufficient to predict continuing abuse [121]; it is probably not enough, therefore, to focus on the alleviation of stress or the reinforcing of coping skills. In all cases where individual and/or family pathology is identified, these should be the object of the initial treatment strategies. Where present, affective disorders, psychoses, alcoholism, and other psychopathology are likely to be making significant contributions to the difficulties in the parent-child interactions. A frontal attack on child abuse is not necessarily the most efficacious or efficient way to deal with it. Ultimately, as *Smith and Rachman* [113] have pointed out, one must change not only parental behaviors but also parental attitudes.

Inducing changes in family patterns of functioning and behavior also appears to be an essential component of most effective treatment programs. Individual, group, and family therapy all have proponents in the field, yet none appears to be better than others. In addition to the more traditional treatments [122], various forms of behavior therapy [113, 123] and self-help groups like Parents Anonymous have proven useful in decreasing abuse [36]. What seems common to all good treatment is that the parents are willing to allow the children to change and to make changes themselves and that the therapist is effective in facilitating the abused child's adaptation to peer and social relationships [124].

Finally, one must attend to the child and his or her individual functioning. Our interest in the child's reactions to the abuse should not make us neglect his or her contribution to the family situation. Children with 'difficult temperaments' [125], for example, are much harder to parent and are more disruptive to family structures. The child's reactions to abusive situations are complex. Children respond differently, depending upon their developmental stage, the chronicity and severity of the maltreatment, prior functioning, and the social supports remaining after the abuse. At first, the child is likely to be fearful of additional harm. Responsible adults, family members, and friends can be quite helpful in the most acute phases of the difficulty. Time and a protective, supportive environment will do much, subsequently, to reduce the sharpness of the distress. It is not uncommon for children to appear quite confused after the abuse has been brought into the open. This confusion is related to the many conflicts which arise from the experience of having been abused or neglected. There is understandable ambivalence about the adults, since they are usually caretakers who have taken advantage of the child. For the child, there is a lack of certainty about whom he or she can turn to in the future. The youngster is also embarrassed over having been abused and feels pity for the adult who is apprehended and, of course, guilt over having exposed the adult to punishment. Finally, one often finds the feeling of shame and low self-esteem. How unworthy must a child be who is abused or neglected by the very persons supposed to care for him or her! When indicated, individual and/or group treatment, in conjunction with family intervention, may be useful. Long-term studies are not as yet available to confirm this clinical impression, however.

The abused child is vulnerable to the vicissitudes of development; he or she merits careful observation and follow-up. Although all children may not need 'treatment', they certainly deserve long-term interest on the part of the medical practitioner. Abused children appear to be at least 'at-risk' for developing later psychopathology and/or social dysfunction. With all of the complexities brought into the open by child abuse, clinicians must take particular care not to generalize too broadly or project their own conflicted feelings onto the child or parent. Our own revulsion over what adults can and do perpetrate on children may lead to responses which make the situation even more difficult for the child. The physician's disdain for the acts should not keep the child from expressing his or her mixture of feelings about the adults who have allegedly committet them. To hate a child's parent is not necessarily to be supportive of the child.

In cases of suspected abuse, labeling may not only inappropriately focus on good versus bad distinctions, but also impose such distinctions as acceptable versus unacceptable, sickness versus health, accountable versus excusable, deviancy versus normalcy, capable versus incapable, and, perhaps, most disturbingly, loving versus hating. If one instead focuses on labeling the family as in need of resources, support, and counseling, more constructive goals may be achieved [20]. We cannot change the past, but a prudent and well-informed medical intervention can help facilitate the child's adaptation to the future.

References

1 Polansky, N.A.; Hally, C.; Polansky, N.: Profile of neglect. A survey of the state of knowledge of child neglect (US Department of Health, Education, and Welfare, Washington 1976).

2 Kalisch, B.J.: Child abuse and neglect. An annotated bibliography (Greenwood Press, Westport 1978).

3 Wells, D.P.: Child abuse. An annotated bibliography (Scarecrow Press, Metuchen 1980).

4 National Institute of Justice. Child abuse and neglect. A literature review and selected bibliography (National Institute of Justice, Washington 1980).

5 Smith, S.L.: Significant research findings in the etiology of child abuse. Social Casework 65: 337–346 (1984).

6 Friedrich, W.N.; Einbender, A.J.: The abused child. A psychological review. J. clin. Child. Psychol. 12: 244–256 (1983).

7 Juvenile Justice Standards Project, Institute of Judicial Administration, American Bar Association: Standards relating to abuse and neglect (Ballinger, Cambridge 1981).

8 Wolock, I.; Horowitz, B.: Child maltreatment as a social problem. The neglect of neglect. Am. J. Orthopsychiat. 54: 530–543 (1984).

9 Fontana, V.: Somewhere a child is crying: maltreatment – its causes and prevention (MacMillan, New York 1973).

10 Gil, D.G.: Violence against children: physical child abuse in the United States (Harvard University Press, Cambridge 1970).

11 Silver, L.B.; Dublin, C.C.; Lourie, R.S.: Child abuse syndrome. The 'gray' areas in establishing a diagnosis. Pediatrics, Springfield 44: 594–600 (1969).

12 Giovannoni, J.; Becerra, R.: Defining child abuse (Free Press, New York 1979).

13 Steele, B.; Pollock, C.: A psychiatric study of parents who abuse infants and small children; in Helfer, Kempe, The battered child, pp. 103–148 (University of Chicago Press, Chicago 1968).

14 Aber, J.L., III; Zigler, E.: Developmental considerations in the definition of child maltreatment; in Rizley, Cicchetti, New directions for child development: developmental perspectives on child maltreatment, pp. 1–29 (Jossey-Bass, San Francisco 1981).

15 Valentine, D.P.; Acuff, D.S.; Freeman, M.L.; et al.: Defining child maltreatment. A multidisciplinary overview. Child Welfare 43: 497–509 (1984).

16 DeFrancis, V.: Child abuse: preview of a nationwide survey (American Humane Association, Denver 1963).

17 Light, R.J.: Abused and neglected children in America. A study of alternative policies. Harvard Educ. Rev. 43: 556–598 (1973).

18 American Association for Protecting Children: Highlights of official child neglect and abuse reporting 1983 (American Humane Association, Denver 1985).

19 National Committee for Prevention of Child Abuse: The size of the child abuse problem, Working Paper 008 (National Committee for Prevention of Child Abuse, Chicago 1985).

20 Reece, R.M.; Grodin, M.A.: Recognition of nonaccidental injury. Pediat. Clins N. Am. 32: 41–60 (1985).

21 Simons, B.; Downs, E.F.; Hurster, M.M.; et al.: Child abuse. Epidemiologic study of medically reported cases. N.Y. St. J. Med. *66:* 2783–2788 (1966).

22 Zuckerman, K.; Ambuel, J.P.; Bandman, R.: Child neglect and abuse. A study of cases evaluated at Columbus Children's Hospital in 1968–1969. Ohio St. med. J. *68:* 629–632 (1972).

23a American Humane Association: Highlights of the 1979 national data (American Humane Association, Englewood 1981).

23b National Center on Child Abuse and Neglect: Study findings. National study of the incidence and severity of child abuse and neglect (National Center on Child Abuse and Neglect, Washington 1981).

24 Ebbin, A.J.; Gollub, M.H.; Stein, A.M.; et al.: Battered child syndrome at the Los Angeles County General Hospital. Am. J. Dis. Child. *118:* 660–667 (1969).

25 Lauer, B.; Ten Broeck, E.; Grossman, M.: Battered child syndrome. Review of 130 patients with controls. Pediatrics, Springfield *54:* 67–70 (1974).

26 Smith, S.M.; Hanson, R.: Interpersonal relationships and childrearing practices in 214 parents of battered children. Br. J. Psychiat. *127:* 513–525 (1975).

27 Gelles, R.J.; Straus, M.A.: Violence in the American family. J. soc. Iss. *35:* 15–39 (1979).

28 Blumberg, M.L.: Depression in abused and neglected children. Am. J. Psychother. *30:* 342–355 (1981).

29 Pagelow, M.D.: Family violence (Praeger, New York 1984).

30 Erlanger, H.S.: Social class differences in parents' use of physical punishment; in Steinmetz, Straus, Violence in the family, pp. 150–158 (Dodd, Mead & Co., New York 1974).

31 Herrenkohl, E.C.; Herrenkohl, R.C.: A comparison of abused children and their non-abused siblings. J. Am. Acad. Child Psychiat. *18:* 260–269 (1979).

32 Sameroff, A.: Transactional models in early social relations. Hum. Devel. *18:* 65–79 (1975).

33 Morse, C.W.; Sahler, O.J.; Friedman, S.B.: A three-year follow-up study of abused and neglected children. Am. J. Dis. Child. *120:* 439–446 (1970).

34 Rosenbloom, L.; Hensey, O.J.: Outcome for children subject to nonaccidental injury. Archs. Dis. Childn. *60:* 191–192 (1985).

35 Pelton, L.H.: Child abuse and neglect. The myth of carelessness. Am. J. Orthopsychiat. *48:* 608–617 (1978).

36 Parke, R.D.; Collmer, C.W.: Child abuse. An interdisciplinary analysis; in Hetherington, Review of child development research, vol. 5., pp. 509–590 (University of Chicago Press, Chicago 1975).

37 Lenington, S.: Child abuse. The limits of sociobiology. Ethol. Sociobiol. *2:* 17–29 (1981).

38 Shearman, J.K.; Evans, E.; Boyle, M.H.; Cuddy, L.J.; Norman, G.R.: Maternal and infant characteristics in abuse. A case control study. J. fam. Pract. *16:* 289–293 (1983).

39 Webster-Stratton, C.: Comparison of abusive and non-abusive families with conduct-disordered children. Am. J. Orthopsychiat. *55:* 59–69 (1985).

40 Elmer, E.; Gregg, G.S.: Developmental characteristics of abused children. Pediatrics, Springfield *40:* 596–602 (1967).

41 Watkins, H.D.; Bradbard, M.R.: Child maltreatment. An overview with suggestions for intervention and research. Fam. Rel. *31:* 323–333 (1982).

42 Martin, H.P.: The abused child. A multidisciplinary approach to developmental issues and treatment (Ballinger, Cambridge 1976).

43 Garbarino, J.A.: The human ecology of child maltreatment: A conceptual model for research. J. Marriage Fam. *1977:* 721–235.

44 Straus, R.; Gelles, R.; Steinmetz, S.: Behind closed doors (Doubleday, New York 1979).

45 Garbarino, J.A.: A preliminary study of ecological correlates of child abuse. The impact of socioeconomic stress on mothers. Child Dev. *47:* 1780–1785 (1976).

46 Garbarino, J.; Sherman, D.: High-risk neighborhoods and high-risk families. The human ecology of child maltreatment. Child Dev. *51:* 188–198 (1980).

47 Holmes, T.; Rahe, R.: The social readjustment rating scale. J. psychosom. Res. *11:* 212–220 (1967).

48 Gourash, N.: Help-seeking. A review of the literature. Am. J. Commun. Psychol. *6:* 413–423 (1978).

49 Lewis, M.: Nearest neighbor analysis of epidemiological and community variables. Psychol. Bull. *85:* 1302–1308 (1978).

50 Dietrich, K.N.; Starr, R.H., Jr.; Weisfeld, G.E.: Infant maltreatment. Caretaker-infant interaction and developmental consequences at different levels of parenting failure. Pediatrics, Springfield *72:* 532–540 (1983).

51 Egeland, B.; Deinard, A.; Brunnquell, D.; et al.: Three and six-month observations of feed and play (University of Minnesota, Minneapolis, unpubl. paper, 1975).

52 Wasserman, G.A.; Green, A.; Allen, R.: Going beyond abuse. Maladaptive patterns of interaction in abusing mother-infant pairs. J. Am. Acad. Child Psychiat. *22:* 245–252 (1983).

53 Fontana, V.J.; Robison, E.: Observing child abuse. J. Pediat. *105:* 655–660 (1984).

54 Blehar, M.C.; Lieberman, A.F.; Ainsworth, M.D.S.: Early face-to-face interaction and its relation to later infant-mother attachment. Child Dev. *48:* 182–184 (1977).

55 Gaensbauer, T.J.; Sands, K.: Distorted affective communications in abused/neglect-ed infants and their potential impact on caretakers. J. Am. Acad. Child Psychiat. *18:* 236–250 (1979).

56 George, C.; Main, M.: Social interactions of young abused children: approach, avoidance, and aggression. Child Dev. *50:* 306–318 (1979).

57 Fraser, B.G.: The child and his parents. A delicate balance of rights; in Helfer, Kempe, Child abuse and neglect: the family and the community, pp. 315–333 (Ballinger, Cambridge 1976).

58 Kempe, C.M.; Silverman, F.N.; Steele, B.F.; et al.: The battered-child syndrome. J. Am. med. Ass. *181:* 17–24 (1962).

59 Heins, M.: The 'battered child' revisited. J. Am. med. Ass. *251:* 3295–3300 (1984).

60 Buchanan, A.; Oliver, J.E.: Abuse and neglect as a cause of mental retardation. A study of 140 children admitted to subnormality hospitals in Wiltshire. Br. J. Psychiat. *131:* 458–467 (1977).

61 Caffey, J.: On the theory and practice of shaking infants. Its potential residual effects of permanent brain damage and mental retardation. Am. J. Dis. Child. *124:* 161–169 (1972).

62 Martin, H.P.: The child and his development; in Hempe, Helfer, Helping the battered child and his family (Lippincott, Philadelphia 1972).

63 Martin, H.P.; Beezley, P.; Conway, E.F.; et al.: The development of abused chil-

dren. I. A review of the literature. II. Physical, neurologic, and intellectual outcome. Adv. Pediat. *21:* 25–73 (1974).

64 Sandgrund, A.; Gaines, R.W.; Green, A.H.: Child abuse and mental retardation: A problem of cause and effect. Am. J. ment. Defic. *79:* 327–330 (1974).

65 Lynch, M.: Risk factors in the child. A study of abused children and their siblings; in Martin, The abused child: a multidisciplinary approach to developmental issues and treatment, pp. 43–56 (Ballinger Press, Cambridge 1976).

66 Hergenroeder, A.C.; Taylor, P.M.; Rogers, K.D.; Taylor, F.H.: Neonatal characteristics of maltreated infants and children. Am. J. Dis. Child. *139:* 295–298 (1985).

67 Leventhal, J.M.; Egerter, S.A.; Murphy, J.M.: Reassessment of the relationship of perinatal risk factors and child abuse. Am. J. Dis. Child. *138.* 1034–1039 (1984).

68 McCabe, V.: Abstract perceptual information for age level. A risk factor for maltreatment. Child Dev. *55:* 267–276 (1984).

69 Gregg, G.S.; Elmer, E.: Infant injuries. Accident or abuse? Pediatrics, Springfield *44:* 434–439 (1969).

70 Sobel, R.: The psychiatric implications of accidental poisoning in childhood. Pediat. Clins N. Am. *17:* 653–685 (1970).

71 Martin, H.P.: The consequences of being abused and neglected: how the child fares; in Kempe, Helfer, The battered child; 3rd ed., pp. 347–365 (University of Chicago Press, Chicago 1980).

72 Zinkus, P.W.; Gottlieb, M.L.; Schapiro, M.: Development and psychoeducational sequelae of chronic otitis media. Am. J. Dis. Child. *132:* 1100–1104 (1978).

73 Lynch, M.A.: The prognosis of child abuse. J. Child Psychol. Psychiat. *19:* 175–180 (1978).

74 Blager, F.; Martin, H.P.: Speech and language of abused children; in Martin, The abused child: a multidisciplinary approach to developmental issues and treatment, pp. 83–92 (Ballinger, Cambridge 1976).

75 Elmer, E.: A follow-up study of traumatized children. Pediatrics, Springfield *59:* 273–279 (1977).

76 Lynch, M.A.; Roberts, J.: Consequences of child abuse (Academic Press, New York 1982).

77 Appelbaum, A.S.: Developmental retardation in infants as an concomitant of physical child abuse. J. abnorm. Child Psychol. *5:* 417–423 (1977).

78 Koski, M.A.; Ingram, E.M.: Child abuse and neglect. Effects on Bayley Scale scores. J. abnorm. Child Psychol. *5:* 79–91 (1977).

79 Dietrich, K.N.; Starr, R.H., Jr.; Kaplan, M.G.: Maternal stimulation and care of abused infants; in Field, High-risk infants and children: adult and peer interactions (Academic Press, New York 1980).

80 Fitch, M.H.; Cadol, R.V.; Goldson, E.; et al.: Cognitive development of abused and failure-to-thrive children. J. pediat. Psychol. *1:* 32–37 (1976).

81 Einbender, A.J.; Friedrich, W.N.: A validation study of the Family Relations Test with physically abused children. Unpublished manuscript, Department of Psychology, University of Washington, Seattle: Cited in Friedrich, W.N.; Einbender, A.J.: The abused child. A psychological review. J. clin. Child Psychol. *12:* 250 (1983).

82 Barahal, R.M.; Waterman, J.; Martin, H.P.: The social cognitive-development of abused children. J. consult. clin. Psychol. *49:* 508–516 (1981).

83 Hoffman-Plotkin, D.; Twentyman, C.T.: A multimodal assessment of behavioral

and cognitive deficits in abused and neglected preschoolers. Child Dev. *55:* 794–802 (1984).

84 Kent, J.T.: A follow-up study of abused children. J. pediat. Psychol. *1:* 25–31 (1976).

85 Martin, H.P.; Beezley, P.: Personality of abused children; in Martin, The abused child: a multidisciplinary approach to developmental issues and treatment, pp. 105–111 (Ballinger, Cambridge 1976).

86 Johnson, B.; Morse, H.: Injured children and their parents. Children *15:* 147–152 (1968).

87 Elmer, E.: Children in jeopardy. A study of abused minors and their families (University of Pittsburgh Press, Pittsburgh 1967).

88 Rolston, R.H.: The effect of prior physical abuse on the expression of overt and fantasy aggressive behavior in children. Diss. Abstr. Int. *32B:* 3016 (1971).

89 Bowlby, J.: Violence in the family as a disorder of the attachment and caregiving systems. Am. J. Psychoanal. *44:* 9–27 (1984).

90 Lewis, D.O.; Shanok, S.S.; Pincus, J.H.; et al.: Violent juvenile delinquents. Psychiatric, neurological, psychological, and abuse factors. J. Am. Acad. Child Psychiat. *18:* 307–319 (1979).

91 Straker, G.; Jacobson, R.S.: Aggression, emotional maladjustment, and empathy in the abused child. Dev. Psychol. *17:* 762–765 (1981).

92 Smetana, J.G.; Kelly, M.; Twentyman, C.T.: Abused, neglected, and maltreated children's conceptions of moral and social-conventional transgressions. Child Div. *55:* 277–287 (1984).

93 Green, A.H.: Psychopathology of abused children. J. Am. Acad. Child Psychiat. *17:* 92–103 (1978).

94 Reidy, T.J.: The aggressive characteristics of abused and neglected children. J. clin. Psychol. *33:* 1140–1145 (1977).

95 Hjorth, C.W.; Harway, M.: The body-image of physically abused and normal adolescents. J. clin. Psychol. *37:* 863–866 (1981).

96 Blain, G.H.; Bergner, R.M.; Lewis, M.L.; et al.: The use of objectively scorable house-tree-person indicators to establish child abuse. J. clin. Psychol. *37:* 667–673 (1981).

97 McCrea, C.W.; Summerfield, A.B.; Rosen, B.: Body image. A selective review of existing measurement techniques. Br. J. med. Psychol. *55:* 225–233 (1982).

98 Hyman, C.A.; Mitchell, R.: A psychological study of child battering. Hth Visitor *48.* 294–296 (1975).

99 Herzberger, S.D.; Potts, D.A.; Dillon, M.A.: Abusive and nonabusive parental treatment from the child's perspective. J. consult. clin. Psychol. *49:* 81–90 (1981).

100 Justice, B.; Justice, R.: The abusing family (Human Sciences Press, New York 1976).

101 Morton, C.: What does the literature say about the correlation between child abuse and juvenile delinquency? (ED204699 ERIC Document Report Service, Arlington 1980).

102 Rogers, S.; LeUnes, A.: A psychometric and behavioral comparison of delinquents who were abused as children with their non-abused peers. J. clin. Psychol. *35:* 470–472 (1979).

103 Fraiberg, S.; Adelson, E.; Shapiro, V.: Ghosts in the nursery. A psychoanalytic

approach to the problems of impaired infant-mother relationships; in Fraiberg, Clinical studies in infant mental health: the first year of life, pp. 164–196 (Basic Books, New York 1980).

104 Fitch, F.J.; Papentonio, A.: Men who batter. Some pertinent characteristics. J. nerv. ment. Dis. *171:* 190–192 (1983).

105 Fagan, J.; McMahon, P.P.: Incipient multiple personality in children. Four cases. J. nerv. ment. Dis. *172:* 26–36 (1984).

106 Greaves, G.: Multiple personality 165 years after Mary Reynolds. J. nerv. ment. Dis. *168:* 577–595 (1980).

107 Solomon, R.S.; Solomon, V.: Differential diagnosis of the multiple personality. Psychol. Rep. *51:* 1187–1194 (1982).

108 Oates, R.K.: Personality development after physical abuse. Archs. Dis. Childn. *59:* 147–150 (1984).

109 Kinard, E.M.: The psychological consequences of abuse for the child. J. soc. Issues *35:* 82–100 (1979).

110 Kinard, E.M.: Emotional development in physically abused children. Am. J. Orthopsychiat. *50:* 686–696 (1980).

111 Feshbach, S.: Aggression; in Mussen, Carmichael's manual of child psychology; 3rd ed., vol. 2, pp. 159–259 (Wiley, New York 1970).

112 Goode, W.J.: Force and violence in the family; in Steinmetz, Strauss, Violence in the family (Dodd, Mead, New York 1974).

113 Smith, J.E.; Rachman, S.J.: Non-accidental injury to children. II. A controlled evaluation of a behavioral management programme. Behav. Res. Ther. *22:* 349–366 (1984).

114 Martin, H.P.; Rodeheffer, M.: Learning and intelligence; in Martin, The abused child: a multidisciplinary approach to developmental issues and treatment, pp. 93–104 (Ballinger, Cambridge 1976).

115 Rohner, R.P.: Parental acceptance-rejection and personality development. A universalist approach to behavorial science; in Brislin, Bochner, Loner, Cross-cultural perspectives on learning (Sage Publications, Bevery Hills 1975).

116 Summit, R.; Kryso, J.: Sexual abuse of children. A clinical spectrum. Am. J. Orthopsychiat. *48:* 237–251 (1978).

117 National Center on Child Abuse and Neglect: A curriculum on the identification, reporting, referral and case management of child abuse and neglect (Children's Bureau, Office of Child Development, US Department of Health, Education, and Welfare, Washington 1976).

118 Newberger, E.H.; Newberger, C.M.; Hampton, R.L.: Child abuse. The current theory base and future research needs. J. Am. Acad. Child. *22:* 262–268 (1983).

119 Smith, J.E.: Non-accidental injury to children. Part I. Behav. Res. Ther. *22:* 331–347 (1984).

120 Cohn, A.H.: Essential elements of successful child abuse and neglect treatment. Child Abuse Neglect *3:* 491–496 (1979).

121 Egeland, B.; Breitenbucher, M.; Rosenberg, D.: Prospective study of the significance of life stress in the etiology of child abuse. J. consult. clin. Psychol. *24:* 195–205 (1980).

122 Green, A.H.: Psychiatric treatment of abused children. J. Am. Acad. Child Psychiat. *17:* 356–371 (1978).

123 Isaacs, C.D.: Treatment of child abuse. A review of the behavioral interventions. J. appl. behav. Anal. *15:* 273–294 (1982).

124 Mrazek, D.; Mrazek, P.: Child maltreatment; in Rutter, Hersov, Child and adolescent psychiatry; 2nd ed., pp. 679–697 (Blackwell, London 1985).

125 Thomas, A.; Chess, S.: Temperament and development (Brunner/Mazel, New York 1977).

Bennet L. Leventhal, MD, Child Psychiatry and Center for Developmental Studies, Department of Psychiatry, The University of Chicago, Chicago, IL 60601 (USA)

II. Behavioral Responses to Trauma

Adv. psychosom. Med., vol. 16, pp. 84–92 (Karger, Basel 1986)

Acute Response to Trauma

Linda G. Peterson

Emergency Mental Health Services, University of Massachusetts Medical Center, Worcester, Mass., USA

Patients who become trauma victims, often have preexisting acute and chronic psychosocial problems. After the trauma, they face additional physical disruption and psychological and social stress. Many factors affect the patient's response to his injury. Physical factors include: (1) overall severity of injury; (2) loss of limbs; (3) loss of sensory organs; (4) presence of brain damage; (5) presence of drugs, alcohol or abstinence syndromes, and (6) complicating medical conditions. Psychological factors include: (1) patient's mental state at time of injury; (2) sense of responsibility for the accident; (3) reaction to injury; (4) reaction to effects on others; (5) degree of memory for the event, and (6) usual coping skills under stress. Social factors include: (1) availability of social support; (2) financial responsibility; (3) legal complications, and (4) loss of significant others.

All of these factors interact to create the observed response to trauma. In the acute phase (which spans the immediate period after injury to the end of hospitalization), physical factors predominate, but these are rapidly modified by psychological and social factors. These shifting parameters require that treatment take into account all three dimensions.

Immediately following trauma, a state of shock or emotional outcry as described by *Horowitz* [1] is seen in most patients. Many patients, however, have received either severe bodily injuries and/or head injuries which impede their ability to process information. For these patients, the first few days to weeks of hospitalization may be a period of confusion with spotty memory resulting from multiple surgeries, general anesthetics, head injuries, and medications which impair per-

Table I. Work-up for delirium in trauma patients

CAT scan – will pick up missed trauma
EEG – differentiates metabolic encephalopathy from focal damage
Review of drug screen and alcohol level from admission
Urine drug screen
Careful drug and alcohol history from family
CBC
SMAC – especially liver functions, BUN, Cr
Mg^{++}
Zn^{++}
Cu^+
Folate level – or based on albumin and protein levels
  automatic effort to improve nutritional status including calorie counts
If fever or increased WBC, cultures
Consider LP

---

ception. Delirium is common during this period. It may be secondary to direct brain injury, drug effects, drug withdrawal, metabolic disturbances, or infection. In victims of motor vehicle accidents (MVA), head trauma is common. Head trauma may be generalized with cerebral edema or localized with contusions, often to the frontal and temporal lobes. Both types of injury affect behavior. The effects may include delirium, dementia, depressive symptoms, amnestic syndromes, and (most commonly in this early period) marked mood and behavioral lability.

Drug effects include the effects of narcotic analgesics, anesthetics, steroids, or other agents which alter the level of consciousness, disturb memory, and alter behavior. Drug withdrawal, most commonly from alcohol, sedative hypnotics, or anxiolytic agents, may appear any time from admission to 2 weeks later. Common metabolic disturbances in this phase include electrolytic imbalances, liver or kidney malfunction, and disturbances due to poor nitritional status with resultant deficiencies of trace metals (Mg, Zn, Cu), vitamins (B complex and especially thiamine) and folate. CNS infections or sepsis may also cause changes in mental status. All of these disturbances produce a wide variety of psychiatric symptoms ranging from anxiety and depression to delirium and frank psychosis. The type of presentation does not imply the etiology; so careful review of history, medications, and laboratory data is needed to reveal the cause (table I). All too often, more than one etiology is present, complicating both assessment and management. The following is a typical example.

   Mr. M. was a 40-year-old married white male engineer in a major corporation who was involved in a motor vehicle accident. He sustained multiple fractures, and a possible frontal lobe contusion. The patient lost consciousness for an unspecified period of time, probably less than 24 h, but since then had been agitated and confused. There was a drinking history of two to three bourbon and waters a night, but no past sequelae of alcohol abuse such as blackouts, gastrointestinal bleeding, shakes, or DTs was noted. He was placed immediately on chlordiazepoxide 75 mg q.i.d., diphenylhydantoin 100 mg t.i.d., acetaminophen and codeine compound one to two tablets every 4 h, and thiamine. On interview several days later, the patient was intermittently somnolent and agitated. He could follow simple commands, but could not give more than one word answers to questions, would give his own name and his wife's, but was otherwise totally disoriented. He could not recall three objects even at one minute and had no memory for recent events. He could not name common objects. At times his speech patterns appeared like those seen in a fluent aphasia. He had no hallucinations or delusions. The patient was felt to have an organic brain syndrome with possible aphasia. Four etiologies were suggested: (1) delirium tremens; (2) head trauma; (3) paradoxical reaction to chlordiazepoxide, or (4) a combination of one and two. Since the patient had shown no improvement on chlordiazepoxide, it was discontinued and the patient was placed on haldoperidol 5 mg every 2 h p.r.n. CT scan at that time showed mild atrophy. EEG showed generalized slowing compatible with a metabolic encephalopathy. All other laboratory tests were normal. Agitation decreased after a week, but the patient continued to have intermittent confusion and confabulation with significant retrograde amnesia. After a month, Mr. M's behavior was moderately improved. He was oriented in three spheres, but still had moderate memory and judgement impairment and was just beginning to comprehend the sequelae of his injury.

   Both alcohol withdrawal and head injury played a role in this case and treating one exacerbated the other, necessitating a change in management. Combinations of etiologies are quite common in these patients. Even after successful correction of such problems, improved mentation may not appear for days to months.

   A four-pronged approach to management is the most effective strategy in treating trauma patients and consists of correcting the underlying medical problem (if possible), psychopharmacologic intervention for immediate symptom relief, discussion with family and staff of the expected course, and use of environmental manipulations to minimize symptoms (table II).

   The two primary pharmacologic agents used are benzodiazepines or neuroleptics. Chlordiezepoxide or diazepam are especially useful in drug withdrawal and with symptoms of anxiety or sleep disturbance in patients *without* cognitive deficit. Short-acting benzodiazepines should be avoided as they may produce withdrawal symptoms unless carefully

Table II. Environmental approaches to delirium

Night light
Frequent orientation cues by nurses, family, etc.
Radio with pleasant background music
Not TV – may cause increased agitation
Sign on wall with doctors names, nurses names, and date
Restraints if necessary

---

titrated. If patients have unrecognized organic deficits, they may have a paradoxical reaction with increased agitation or even psychotic behavior when given benzodiazepines, in which case the patient should be switched to a neuroleptic. Neuroleptics are advocated if cognitive deficit or significant delusional or hallucinatory experience is present. Neuroleptic or antipsychotic agents that are most useful for these patients are haloperidol (haldol) and trifluperazine (trilafon). These agents can be used intravenously, intramuscularly, and orally. They have a low anticholinergic profile, so they will not interact with anticholinergic agents used to potentiate narcotics or used preoperatively. Trifluperazine will itself potentiate narcotic analgesics and haloperidol may have a similar effect. Trifluperazine also acts as an antiemetic agent and appetite stimulant, two properties which may be helpful in a trauma patient. Generally low doses (1–5 mg) are adequate to decrease agitation, hallucinations, and delusions, although some patients may require a typical antipsychotic dose (5–30 mg). Use of these agents intravenously has the additional advantage of minimal or no extrapyramidal effects. Laryngospasm may occur if used intravenously, but can be reversed with epinephrine [2].

Environmental support at this time should include frequent orientation to time and place, reassurance that these symptoms will resolve, use of radio and night lights to diminish 'sundowning', and repeated, careful explanations of all procedures to the patient. As cognitive functioning, memory, and concentration improve, patients will begin to respond to their physical and emotional losses. This may occur all at once or in stages. Those patients with the least physical impairment will arrive at this stage most rapidly and are more likely to have a stage of shock or emotional outcry. Patients may be more likely to develop post-traumatic stress disorders if they retained consciousness during the original event. Patients with less physical impairment and unimpaired memory will be reacting to their losses at the same time others involved in the event and uninvolved family and friends. This will give them the opportunity to share feelings of loss, anger, sadness, and pain which will facilitate their psychological recovery. Patients who understand the nature of their losses days to weeks later will enter the grieving process at a different stage than their family and friends. This may cause increased strain in communication. For example, the family may become very protective and feel unsure how much to reveal to the patient for fear of affecting their physical recovery. This may make the patient feel left out and even more dependent and helpless. The family needs encouragement and support to share 'bad news' with the patient and cope with the emotional response of the patient. Also in patients who are alert, but likely to have prolonged hospitalizations because of burns, multiple fractures or other complications, the family should be encouraged to include the patient in handling day to day affairs they would normally have controlled. Patients need to be given as much of an active role as they can handle to improve their self-esteem and encourage their most effective coping skills.

Nurses may often be distressed by sudden emotional outbursts in patients who have been quiet and tractable while their mentation was impaired. It is essential to educate nursing staff about the emotional upheaval that may follow realization of deficits in these patients and to help them support healthy verbalization and emotional display of distress. Techniques of brief supportive intervention will assist nurses in feeling comfortable dealing with these patients' emotional distress and make them effective in promoting psychological recovery of the patients.

The following case is illustrative of the intermediate phase:

Mrs. B. was a 30-year-old married white female nurse who was in a serious motorcycle accident 3 weeks prior to consultation. Her husband was killed in the same accident. Mrs. B. suffered head trauma and had no memory of the accident. She knew that her husband was dead and that he was still unburied in a funeral home in another town. She had avoided, deliberately, talking about her husband, because she had been afraid that she would 'lose her mind'. The day prior to consultation, she decided that she was making herself worse by trying to avoid grieving, so she asked to see a psychiatrist. She stated she was ready to start talking about her husband's death and let herself grieve. In spite of this statement, Mrs. B. was only intermittently willing to talk about her husband. She often refused to continue, saying that talking about him made her headaches worse. On several occasions, she spent hours crying which she later recognized as related to grief for her husband and her own physical losses. At other times, she had fights with the nurses over trivial matters. She realized later that her losses made her resent the healthy nurses who took care of her. Even after her discharge, her ability to deal with grief was sporadic for several months after injury.

In several similar cases, patients who remained for a prolonged period in this state of numbness often felt that they were personally responsible for the death or disability of others involved in the accident, whether this was realistic or not. Mrs. B., for example, felt that she was responsible for her husband's death, because she asked him to take her to visit a patient, since her car was not running. During this period, problems with dreams of the accident or other distressing feelings about the event are common. At times, if sleep disturbance and post-traumatic dreaming is excessive, low dose tricyclic antidepressant medication (imipramine 25–50 mg q.h.s.) may improve sleep and allow better verbalization of grief. Most patients after several weeks pass through this phase into one of oscillating depression and anger.

Some patients will have predominantly angry responses, depending on the traumatic event, previous personality traits and responses to stress in the past. In fact, one study of trauma patients found significantly more hostility among these patients than other groups of hospitalized patients [3]. Others may appear primarily depressed and sad. Key factors in this stage are the duration of hospitalization, degree of disability, other losses suffered during the traumatic event and amount of emotional support available from staff, family, and friends. Some patients are particularly angry because they are the victims of the carelessness of a drunk driver and feel no control over their injury. Depression is most common among patients who have been hospitalized a long time with ambiguous prognoses which are continuously being revised. Often they have had repeated surgeries over a period of months to years and are unclear about whether they will ever fully recover.

Mr. L. was a 27-year-old married white male, whose wife was killed in the accident in which his own leg was crushed. Mr. L. was sleeping in the back of the station wagon at the time of the accident. He was pinned by his injury, but could hear the driver of the other vehicle saying (about his wife) 'Oh my God, she's dead.' With multiple grafts, use of a Hoffman device, and several other surgeries, an attempt was made to save his leg resulting in over six lengthy hospitalizations in the subsequent year. Initially, Mr. L. asked to see a psychiatrist to talk about his anger over his wife's death and the careless driver responsible. He also was concerned about his leg. He described some past difficulty with drug abuse when in military service and was worried that he would cope with his fears by abusing drugs. Several hospitalizations later the question of viability of his leg became less clear, by then he had been bedridden for over 6 months. He began to be abusive to the staff, often threatening to leave against medical advice, demanding drugs and stating that he did not care if he was addicted. After his amputation below the knee 1 year later, he returned to work and school and has had no further emotional problems.

Mr. L. suffered anger early on, because of his sense of being injured and losing his wife due to the other driver's carelessness and intoxication. He also felt helpless because of his inability to protect his wife and his lack of control over his medical care. Talking about these feelings allowed him to find ways he could cope with them more effectively. Even after crossing that hurdle, his continued disability, unclear prognosis and lack of available social support caused increased emotional distress and regression to less effective coping. From a psychological point of view, earlier amputation would probably have averted much of the subsequently observed turmoil. This underlines one of the key issues for many trauma patients which is prolonged dependency and ambiguity of outcome. This combination, coupled with grief over other losses, tends to lead patients to regress and demonstrate their most primitive coping skills. This usually alienates them from the hospital staff who must care for them and results in deterioration of care. For these patients, case conferences with nursing staff and family helps to increase tolerance while encouraging more healthy coping styles by the patient. These supportive activities may be critical to minimizing psychological morbidity.

At any time during the recovery from trauma, symptoms of post-traumatic stress disorders may emerge. These need to be distinguished from anxiety, depression or psychotic states. Typically, the patient with post-traumatic stress disorder will report dreams and/or daytime hallucinatory experiences during which they relive the accident. They not only see it happening, but experience overwhelming emotions at the same time including fearfulness, anxiety, rage, helplessness. Along with this, the patient may show diminished interest in rehabilitative activities, seem less accessible to friends and family, and even appear rather emotionless in conversation. Some patients will actively avoid talking about things which remind them of the accident, as these may provoke undesired responses. They may complain about sleep disturbance, memory impairment and difficulty concentrating. They may have an exaggerated startle response or generalized hyperalertness. The key to treatment is reassurance about the normalcy of response to patient, family, and staff. Brief discussions of the event, focussing on connecting feelings with events when not in an oneiric state and possibly use of a short-term (2–3 weeks) low dose (25–30 mg) antidepressant (imipramine) or MAO inhibitor (phenelzine 15–30 mg) may help to decrease anxiety and sleep disturbance. If depressive symptoms continue, increasing the antidepressant to therapeutic levels (imipramine 100–200 mg) and standard course of treatment (4–6 months) should be considered. Often effective treatment of post-traumatic stress disorder will improve the patient's coping skills and allow them to progress more rapidly in both physical and psychological rehabilitation.

Toward the end of hospitalization, patients begin to shift the focus of their attention from physical recovery per se, to their return to home and/or work. Anticipation of how resultant disabilities will affect their function and the reaction of others to them come into play. Also, loss of family members will have to be faced at home including seeing pictures, dealing with the clothes and belongings, and being home without the dead family member for the first time. For patients who generally experience anticipatory anxiety, this part of recovery may be associated with psychological distress and often increased complaints about physical symptoms when discharge appears imminent. These patients can be helped significantly by counselling during the discharge process, discussing alternative approaches to coping, reinforcing their competence to handle these events, and identifying the availability of further counselling if necessary. Brief visits home prior to discharge may also facilitate the final return. Groups for these patients and their families, which they may join shortly before discharge, may provide a safe environment for dealing with the multiple stresses of returning to home and work for the recovering trauma patient.

In summary, when working with patients who are trauma victims, careful attention must be paid to the particular configuration and stage of their psychological response post-trauma, the presence of grief reactions, the response to injury, the presence of preexisting psychiatric problems (particularly alcoholism or depression), the degree of responsibility felt over the traumatic event, the complications that will ensue from the event, and, finally, the potential recovery and support available from family and friends throughout the recovery period. The approaches outlined for dealing with post-traumatic stress disorders based on personality style, and for intervention in patients experiencing acute grief are important tools in working with trauma patients.

References

1 Horowitz, M.J.: Stress response syndromes. Archs gen. Psychiat. *31:* 768–780 (1974).
2 Dudley, D.L.; Rowlett, D.B.; Loebel, P.J.: Emergency use of intravenous haloperidol. Gen. Hosp. Psychiat. *1:* 240–246 (1979).
3 Kane, M.: Hostility reactions in trauma patients; thesis, Texas Women's University, Denton (1977).

Linda G. Peterson, MD, Emergency Mental Health Services, University of Massachusetts Medical Center, Worcester, MA 01605 (USA)

Adv. psychosom. Med., vol. 16, pp. 93–114 (Karger, Basel 1986)

Grief Response in Trauma Patients and Their Families

J. Trig Brown[1]

Division of General Internal Medicine, Duke University Medical Center, Durham, N.C., USA

Introduction

On the morning of Tuesday, January 18, 1977, a disaster occurred at Granville, an outer suburb of Sydney, Australia. A loaded train carrying commuters to work came off the rails and hit a road bridge which collapsed on several carriages. The tragedy was heightened because of the fact that many of the victims and the injured were trapped for many hours under the tonnage of a giant concrete slab from the bridge while rescuers worked frantically to raise this so that they could be freed. The relatives of those trapped under the slab lived with uncertainty for the 36 h that it took to remove the last victim. When the final count was made, 83 people had been killed and about the same number injured [1].

As described above, trauma can result in losses which touch victims, injured, rescuers, and relatives simultaneously. The individual involved in an accident may survive the initial trauma only to be faced with living without certain body parts, bodily functions, or loved ones. Family members and friends of those involved in accidents may suddenly and without warning find themselves thrust into a social structure dramatically changed.

Grief reactions are normal and necessary consequences of these losses. Successful rehabilitation involves the trauma victim grieving the losses imposed by the accident. Family and friends of those killed in accidents must relinquish the ties to their lost loved ones in order to form relationships in the future. Facilitation of this grief response should be included in the comprehensive management of trauma victims.

[1] Dr. *Brown* is funded by the American College of Physicians as a Teaching and Research Scholar.

Medical personnel managing the victims of trauma and interacting with their families and friends are in a prime position to promote normal grieving, evaluate abnormal responses and make referrals for management when appropriate. Many of the psychological responses felt in the trauma victim are mirrored in and felt by these medical personnel. In this way, the effects of trauma span beyond the victim and victim's family and into the lives of the helpers.

In this chapter, grief responses initiated by trauma will be discussed. The trauma victim's response, the families' reactions, and the repercussions for the helpers will be detailed with particular emphasis on facilitating the normal response and recognizing the abnormal reaction. A final section will discuss reactions to civil disasters, circumstances which have some parallels to individual grief responses but also have unique considerations.

Grief Reactions in the Trauma Victim

Normal Reactions

Survival following trauma is often only the first hurdle in recovering from an accident. Depending on the extent and nature of the bodily damage, the trauma may result in significant losses, e.g. loss of body parts, bodily function, independence, personal property. Just as the loss of a loved one precipitates a grief reaction, any significant loss resulting from an accident will be grieved [2].

The grief reaction following injury is adaptive. Through this process the patient examines his life from many angles; where he has been, where he is going, and what goals will not now be met as a result of the injury. A normal grief reaction allows the individual to work through these losses reaching an adaptive conclusion [3]. Success depends upon the passage of time, a sequence of adaptive emotional responses, and a pre-existing state fertile to the healing process. These will be discussed in detail since interference with these negatively influences outcome.

Reactive Stage

The emotional responses of the grief reaction following trauma parallel the phases of physiologic convalescence (table I) [4]. Much of this has been reviewed in the earlier chapter by Dr. *Peterson,* but a brief

Table I. The phases of injury

Phase	Stage of grief	Purpose	Affect
Acute	reactive	protective	absent
			constricted
Convalescent			
	adaptive	acceptance	anger
			hostility
Rehabilitation			dysphoria

review will help clarify later stages. The first emotional stage is called the reactive stage and correlates with the acute phase of injury. This period is dominated by *defensive coping mechanisms* as the trauma victim struggles for life. Repression, denial, reaction formation, regression, projection, displacement and isolation are all employed to prevent the overwhelming aspects of the injury from being realized at the conscious level [5, 6].

Denial, one of the most commonly used adaptive responses, may take on a variety of forms. Rarely, the injury itself will be denied; however, most commonly the importance of the injury, the implications of the injury, and the permanence of the injury are denied [4, 7]. During this first stage, denial is protective; however, later in the course of adaptation denial can significantly interfere with rehabilitation [5].

Affective responses during this stage also stress basic protection. Absent affect with a seemingly resigned attitude can be striking in the face of profound injuries [4]. Although all the specifics of an accident might be discussed in detail during this phase it is usually done with a blunted and constricted affect; thus, further protecting the patient from experiencing the painful emotions following trauma.

Providing for the physiologic needs is the first step in meeting the emotional needs during this reactive stage, the basic management premise must by necessity emphasize stabilizing the patient. The denial is expected, protective, and should not be confronted at this time. As a result of the constriction of the affect, there will be a tendency for the patient to withdraw. This withdrawal is unavoidable but communication channels should be established and clear explanations of all procedures should be routine [7]. Gradually the components of the reactive stage will wane as the patient progresses through their grief work.

Adaptive Stage

The second emotional stage following injury is the *adaptive stage* and spans the final two phases of injury, the convalescent and reha-bilitation phases. During the adaptive stage, the titanic changes im-posed by the injury are assimilated. To adapt to these changes, new patterns of behavior are developed [5, 8, 19].

This stage is often heralded by the surfacing of anger or hostility, signs that the denial is waning [7]. The anger may be projected outward to the staff and family or expressed less directly via rebellion or non-cooperation. Either way, its presence is a sign that the patient is addressing necessary issues on the path to final acceptance and should be encouraged [5]. One method of encouragement involves eliciting a description of the accident and circumstances leading up to it. By discussing this affect-laden area, ventilation of anger and hostility is facilitated, the implications of the injury to the patient are aired, and the patient can be helped to face the realities of the present situation [7, 9].

Dysphoric moods likewise signify an erosion of protective denial. Depending upon the nature of the injury and disability, feelings of shame, self-aversion, expectation of rejection, sense of worthlessness, hopelessness, and helplessness surface. The grief work is painful while the victim is faced with 'the loss of his life as he knew it while yet continuing to live' [7]. However, prolonged depressive episodes are rare.

A good physician-patient relationship has been noted to decrease the depression after spinal cord trauma [5]. Caregivers must examine the ambivalent feelings that surface in themselves as a result of being in the position of caring for the patient but at the same time encourag-ing independence in the patient. By avoiding over-indulgence and excess sympathy, the patient can be approached from an empathic position without fostering regression and dependence [5, 10]. Interac-tions with other patients and staff mobilize hope, reduce isolation, offer group sanction, promote acceptance of the patient as a full person, and thus restore self-esteem [4, 7].

Adaptive mechanisms and affective responses are necessary to facilitate recovery. Gradually helplessness, hopelessness, and despair decrease. The patient learns that life after injury can be rewarding; which preserves his self-esteem. Finally, interpersonal relationships are restored and grief work is completed.

Abnormal Reactions

Just as the original trauma can be complicated by further physiologic derangements, the grief response following injury can have additional complications. Knowledge of abnormal responses to trauma has been gained by observing patients following acute spinal cord injury. Of course the ultimate outcome will be affected greatly by the nature of the injury and the guidelines drawn from the spinal cord literature may not necessarily apply across the board to injuries of different types.

The abnormal grief reactions described are: (1) depressive reactions; (2) psychotic reactions; (3) indifferent reactions; (4) excessive anxiety, and (5) excessive dependency [4, 5, 11, 12].

The frequency of the various types is unknown. 'Depression' is seen in 45% of soldiers in the first 6 months following traumatic paraplegia [13]; however, this figure most likely represents the 'dysphoria' characteristic of the normal reaction to injury and true depressions are rarer [4, 11]. Depressions occurring in the second 6-month period following spinal cord trauma are uncommon and carry a poor prognostic implication [5]. Seventy percent of the survivors of the Coconut Grove nightclub fire disaster had no neuropsychiatric complications [12]. Depressions were rare; however, the following case nicely exemplifies an abnormal reaction with both depressive and excessive anxiety components. .

A youth of 20, a clerk, had been somewhat excitable and easily angered prior to his injury but aside from that had been well adjusted to his professional and married life. On the night of the disaster he was about to leave the night club and stood near an exit waiting for his wife, who was 4 months pregnant. He suddenly saw flames, was milled around, lost sight of his wife and soon escaped through an exit. The patient suffered second degree burns of the face, neck and hands. Five percent of the total skin area was involved. Shortly before leaving the hospital on December 15, 1942, he was told by the priest that his wife had perished in the fire. Until then he had thought she had been saved. He became deeply depressed and has been so ever since. He went back to work in January 1943, but his working capacity has suffered. He is much slower and has lost all interest in his work. In his spare time he thinks of the disaster and of his wife, feels that he will never be interested in another girl. He cannot concentrate and starts shaking all over whenever he has a slight argument. He is constantly afraid of another fire and would never dare to go to a night club again. He sits down in moving pictures only if there is a seat in the last row, so that he can get out quickly. He takes the same precautions in dining rooms. The sound of fire engines awakes him at night with a start. He had had no nightmares in the hospital, but they began 1 week after he came home. In the following months he relived the scenes of the fire in five terrifying dreams. They still occur, though rarely. He had the last nightmare in September 1943. The patient was rejected by the

Army in March 1943 with the diagnosis of psychoneurosis. This depresses him deeply
because he had hoped to be able to forget through strenuous army life. He is trying again
to join the Army and intends to join the Merchant Marine if again rejected [12].

Psychotic reactions are even more unusual. During the acute phase
of injury, hallucinations and delusions may occur but often represent
acute metabolic derangements secondary to the injury. In the Coconut
Grove fire, only two survivors developed psychotic reactions and in
each the history showed clear cut previous maladjustment [4]. Similar
results are reported in survivors of acute spinal cord injury [5].

Nagler [11] describes the third type of abnormal reaction, the
indifferent reaction. These patients exhibit prolonged and complete
hopelessness. They are indifferent, passive and show no motivation to
participate in the rehabilitation program. Theoretically this group is
viewed as suffering reactive depression and are directing their anger
into passivity rather than toward a potentially more dangerous target,
themselves or others. It is suggested that these patients were passive and
dependent before the trauma [15].

Excessive anxiety was the most common abnormal reaction in the
survivors of the Coconut Grove fire. Of the survivors interviewed, 55%
at 3 months and 30% at 9 months had symptoms which would now be
consistent with the diagnosis, generalized anxiety disorder. One-third
of all survivors had nightmares in which the fire was re-experienced
during the hospitalization; however, recurrent nightmares or nightmares beginning weeks after the event correlated with subsequently
developing excessive anxiety. Interestingly, although half the survivors
lost relatives or friends in the fire, this fact seemed to have no effect on
the ultimate outcome [12].

Excessive dependency can follow trauma especially when a permanent disability ensues. During the acute phase of injury, dependency
is a necessary adaptation to reestablish homeostasis; however, during
the convalescent and rehabilitation phases it is maladaptive. This reaction may be manifested by overdependence on the staff, family, medications, alcohol, or as fears of trying new tasks [5]. On the other hand,
'pseudo-independent behavior, e.g. inappropriate confidence, ob-
stinacy, and inability to accept help, can also be a manifestation of this
dependency-independency conflict.

Can the outcome be predicted: Of course the answer is no; however, certain variables do seem correlated with certain outcomes [5, 10,
13]. Healthy premorbid personality development correlates with a bet-

ter outcome. Those victims who were successful, extroverted, and able to delay gratification seem to adjust better than those who were ambitious and impulsive before the trauma. The support network also appears to influence adaptation with those patients having a stable, close-knit family seeming to do better. It appears especially important that the victim feels a firm sense of belonging in the supportive relationship [5]. The data concerning the nature of the accident, intellectual abilities, and economic factors is less understood. Clearly, more research is required in this area.

The Trauma Victim's Family: Grief Response

As the trauma elicits a series of emotional reactions in the victim, the victim's family is also affected. Knowledge of the grief reaction will help medical personnel interacting with the family of those injured. Additionally, these personnel are often bearing the news, informing the family of a death; thus, understanding acute grief reactions is imperative. The family's reactions to the injured and the killed relative will be discussed in the following sections.

The Injured Patient: Family's Reaction

The affective responses the trauma victim experiences are often mirrored in and felt by those around the patient, i.e. the family and staff [16]. During the acute phase of injury, as the victim is employing defensive mechanisms to keep the reality of the situation from consciousness, the family likewise is coping with enormous shock. Their numbed and helpless feelings are only magnified as they are separated from the patient by the many technological devices necessary to restore the physiologic homeostasis. Well-trained staff must meet each vital need for the patient as the family observes from a seemingly helpless posture. Excessive hovering or, oppositely, fleeing by the family can be evidence that the panic has been overwhelming. During this reactive stage of grief the family also readily accepts denial as a defensive maneuver.

The family's needs can be addressed during this stage by providing various active avenues of communication to decrease the family's sense of isolation. An arena for the family to express their feelings of helplessness should be provided and they should be involved in making decisions when possible and encouraged to assist with concrete tasks, e.g.

necessary paper work, mobilizing and communicating with other family and friends, seeing that some of the victim's prior responsibilities are met, etc. Just as in treating the victim, it should be recognized that the denial is protective and should not be too quickly confronted unless it is interfering with treatment.

The victim's anger during the adaptive stage of grief is often targeted towards the family which results in their own guilt, anger and irritability. Explaining the normalcy of these reactions and allowing the families to ventilate their own hostile feelings can go far to defuse this situation.

Initially trauma victims satisfy all of Parsons' sick-role criteria [17]; they are not responsible for their dysfunction because it is beyond their control; since it is beyond their control they are exempt from normal social role responsibilities; they are expected to recognize that the dysfunction is undesirable and are obligated to try to get well; and they are expected to seek appropriate help to get well. From the family, this results in kindness and solicitude. Later during the convalescent and rehabilitation phases of injury, the family's reactions depend greatly upon their perception of the victim's progress [5]. If they view the patient as failing any of the responsibilities of the sick-role, i.e. not trying to get out of the sick-role, resentment can follow. In which case, intervention must be directed at airing expectations, ventilating the feelings aroused by them, and helping both family and patient set realistic goals.

Death From Trauma: Family's Reaction

Loss of a loved one through death most distinctly precipitates a grief reaction. Historically it is through observing relatives of trauma victims that our present understanding of the grief reaction has been formulated. Lindemann's observations of survivors and relatives of those lost in the Coconut Grove Nightclub fire [12, 14, 18, 19] and *Raphael's* [1, 9] interventions with those who lost family members in the Granville Rail Disaster serve as conceptual frameworks upon which most models of grief reaction are built.

Are these models of 'normal' grief reactions? Can we even go so far as to generalize that any one reaction to such tremendous stresses is normal as opposed to outcome. Any series of responses which reaches an adaptive end allowing the individual to extricate himself from the lost person and to reform emotional involvement in new relationships is normal [20]. There are certain feature characteristics of adaptive reactions and these will be elaborated [2]. It should be emphasized that these normal features can be changed in intensity and duration, and the final result can be maladaptive. Later in this section the factors influencing the outcome of grief will be outlined and finally, characteristic types of abnormal reactions will be discussed.

Normal Reactions

Hearing the news of a death of a friend or relative initiates a series of somatic symptoms, mood changes, and behavioral responses which collectively represent the grief reaction. Just as the individual's reaction to trauma has a phasic course, so too can the course of bereavement be conceptionalized [2]. The first phase of the grief reaction is variably termed the phase of shock, protest, denial, or numbness. Most characteristics of this phase is the blunted, numb affect which can be preceded by feelings of tremendous distress.

'I suddenly burst. I was aware of a horrible wailing and knew it was me. I was saying I loved him and all that. I knew he'd gone but I kept talking to him.' She went to the bathroom and retched. Then the feeling of numbness set in. 'I felt numb and solid for a week. It's a blessing. . . Everything goes hard inside you. . . like a heavy weight.' She felt that the numbness enabled her to cope without weeping [21].

The individual may sit motionless, appear dazed, and feel that every movement is made against incredible forces of inertia [22]. A sense of disbelief or unreality predominates as the protective denial keeps the reality of the loss from awareness [21, 23]. As this network of denial is penetrated a definite syndrome of somatic responses appears.

Sensations of somatic distress occuring in waves lasting from 20 min to an hour at a time, a feeling of tightness in the throat, choking with shortness of breath, need for sighing, and an empty feeling in the abdomen, lack of muscular power, and an intense subjective distress described as tension or mental pain [19].

Individuals during this phase require comfort and support. Fear and anxieties must be allowed to be expressed. Sedatives are to be avoided but if the anxieties need temporary reduction, a small amount of sedative for 1 or 2 nights only is usually adequate [9]. Later in this phase the family members should be allowed and encouraged to view the body. This helps to confirm the reality of the death and gives the family an opportunity to say goodbye [20].

As the sense of unreality wanes, the individual enters the second stage of grief, the stage of preoccupation. *Parkes* [21] states that pining for the deceased, so characteristic of this stage, is pathognomonic of the grieving process. Thoughts of the deceased fill the minds of the be-reaved. In an almost ruminative nature, the bereaved focuses on memories of the lost relative, objects in the environment with sentimental meanings, and places shared during the relationship. Recollections of the deceased take on vivid clarity; in fact, over half of the bereaved in one series had frequent dreams of the deceased and many had hallucinations [21].

The numbed affect of the first stage is replaced by anger, guilt, and sadness. Somatic symptoms are frequent and insomnia, anorexia with weight loss, crying and difficulty with concentration predominate [24]. During this stage the bereaved person withdraws and expresses little interest in previous activities. Those people with histories of prior heavy alcohol intake increase their usage during this stage, although there is no increase in those who use it only moderately [24, see article by *Reilly* et al., this vol.].

It is during this second stage that most of the progress towards freeing the individual of previous ties to the deceased takes place and the goal of the medical personnel during this stage is to facilitate this process. Within the framework of the physician-patient relationship the bereaved individual can be gently encouraged to continue this 'relationship review' even in the face of painful affects. To open areas for discussion one can ask questions about the actual circumstances leading up to and including the death, funeral and subsequent time. Follow up questions should inquire about the nature of the relationship with the deceased. Both good and bad memories should be elicited and the affects which ensue should be supported [9, 20, 25, 26].

How long does this process take? There is no uniform agreement. *Clayton* et al. [24] who view the course of uncomplicated grief as relatively benign, found most bereaved improved 6–10 weeks following the loss. On the other hand, *Zisook* et al. [27] noted that grief-related dysphoria peaked between 1 and 2 years after the loss. Additionally, 10 years following the loss, the majority of their sample positively endorsed those items reflecting grief-related feelings: (a) no one will ever take his/her place in my life; (b) I very much miss the person; (c) I've never known a better person; (d) sometimes I dream about him/her [27]. Although the vast majority reported that they were functioning just as well 10 years after as they had before the loss, one-quarter admitted painful memories, crying when they thought about the person, and being upset at the anniversary of the death.

This pining fades into the stage of resolution as the preoccupation with the deceased decreases. Memories of the deceased are still clear but they are now associated with less painful affects. Somatic symptoms decrease, interest in previous activities is rekindled, and the tendency toward social isolation reverses as the individual is now free to form new emotional attachments.

Factors Influencing the Outcome of Grief

Many factors are purported to influence the course of grieving. The following list is a compilation from a number of sources [19, 20, 26, 28–30]:

The Nature of the Relationship before the Loss. If the bereaved individual was dependent upon the lost one, the prognosis for an uncomplicated grief response is said to be poorer. Likewise, if the relationship was characterized by marked ambivalence, the guilt and anger invariably experienced will serve as strong deterrents to working through the second stage of grief. Parents losing children have a poorer outcome in general than other relationships. This undoubtedly reflects the universal guilt feelings aroused within the parent when a child is lost.

The Nature of the Loss Itself. Being able to expect the death helps by allowing some of the grief work to be accomplished before the loss. Unexpected death or death following a relatively brief terminal illness does not allow this anticipatory grief work and thus portends a more protracted mourning. Death following suicide is difficult to mourn for similar reasons and also because of the tremendous amounts of guilt and anger aroused by the suicide.

Social Support Network. Higher socioeconomic status predicts a better prognosis. As *Raphael* [9] has nicely shown, a nonsupportive social network can inhibit the expression of certain affects: 'I felt guilty and when I mentioned that, my family said I shouldn't'; 'I felt angry but my family said it was wrong to feel that way'.

Concurrent Events. Multiple other crises at the time of the loss impedes the normal phasic expression of grief. Similarly, the health of the mourner at the time of the loss is said to have a positive correlation with outcome.

How many of these factors have absolutely been shown to affect the outcome of bereavement? Except for one outstanding study there is really a dearth of prospective data to answer this question. The Granville Train Disaster allowed *Singh and Raphael* [28] to predict outcome based on earlier observations and see if this correlated with the measured outcome. Neither additional crises at the time of the disaster nor ambivalence in the relationship with the deceased predicted eventual outcome. Three factors were predictive of outcome: (a) the relation to the deceased; (b) perception of social network, and (c) viewing the body.

In their study, outcome was measured by a number of techniques 13 months following the disaster. Bereaved spouses did better than bereaved parents and widowers tended to do better than widows. The percentages of bad outcomes are 82, 63, 25, and 22 for mothers, fathers, widows, and widowers, respectively. Most of these parents were beyond the child-bearing age suggesting that emotional replacement of the lost child is more difficult than replacing a lost spouse.

The adequacy of the social network was evaluated at the time of the disaster by an investigator not involved in obtaining the follow-up data. Knowledge of the social network easily predicted outcome. In 80% of those with an adequate network the outcome was good compared to a good outcome in only 40% of those whose network was inadequate.

Many people who lost relatives in this rail disaster elected to not view the body for one reason or another. Of those who viewed the body 75% had a good outcome, only half of those who did not view the body had a good outcome. Only one person who viewed the body regretted it, however, 60% of those who did not view the body expressed regret in having not done so. This, compiled with the outcome data, supports the guideline that relatives should be encouraged to view bodies even following disfiguring accidents.

Abnormal Reactions

The grief response is abnormal if it does not reach the adaptive end. Abnormal responses may be *absent, delayed, blocked,* or *distorted.* The mechanism underlying absent, delayed, and blocked responses is similar and represents either a failure to initiate the grief response or a premature interruption of it because the affects experienced are too painful to deal with on a conscious level [19, 20, 26]. Often the person who fails to initiate a grief reaction is the person who feels responsible for supporting the other family members or is undergoing multiple other crises at the time of the loss. Inability to visit the grave may be a manifestation of absent grieving and may serve the purpose of denying the finality of the loss.

The grief reaction may be interrupted at any point in the sequence resulting in a blocked reaction. During the second stage of grief the bereaved sorts through old memories and a behavioral parallel of this is the sorting through of the deceased's clothing, business articles, etc. The history that things have been left 'just the way they used to be' should suggest a blocked and therefore incomplete grief reaction. Partial blocking of the grief reaction may occur resulting from idealization of the deceased, one has difficulty grieving the total (and thus, real) person if the negative attributes are not allowed expression [26].

Lindemann [19] described nine forms of *distorted* grief reactions: (1) overactivity without a sense of loss; (2) acquisition of symptoms from the deceased's last illness; (3) medical illness; (4) social isolation; (5) hostility towards a specific person; (6) wooden, 'schizophreniform' behavior; (7) loss of social interactions; (8) actions detrimental to their social and economic existence, and (9) agitated depression.

Anger and guilt are often at the root of these disturbed reactions. Management usually requires supportive psychotherapy which encourages the bereaved to specifically explore the death, relationship with the deceased, and the underlying affects.

The morbidity and mortality of the bereaved deserves special mention. Numerous retrospective and prospective studies have addressed this item and varying conclusions have resulted [21, 25, 31–37]. It appears that in the younger bereaved individuals, somatic symptoms, depressive symptoms, and the usage of medications is greater than in age-matched nonbereaved controls. Mortality data is even more variable but it appears that there might be an excessive mortality in elderly widowers especially within the first six months following the loss.

Does the Helper Become the Victim?

Just as the emotional component of the victim's grief reaction can be mirrored in the family, so too are they felt by the staff. The preparation of people helping trauma victims varies and fills a spectrum from no training (the volunteer who spontaneously stops to help) to sharply honed intensive care training (i.e. the surgical intensive care unit staff). The training of most helpers falls somewhere in the middle of these two extremes. Regardless of the training, interactions during emotionally highly charged times affect all and should be addressed at some time during or following the crises.

The first reactions described by helpers is also that of shock, disbelief and a sense of unreality [1, 9, 16]. These defensive reactions enable the helpers to function despite the enormous stresses. A 'split' functioning is described with the helper able to carry out tasks effortlessly without exhaustion but not reacting emotionally to the distressing events surrounding them. This sets the stage for a delayed expression of these experienced emotions.

If the helper feels adequately trained and is able to perform the needed tasks, a very positive, assured, heightened involvement may surface. There may be an over involvement with a reluctance to allow other adequately trained helpers to take over. On the other hand, if the helper is unable to perform the needed acts or feels inadequately prepared, feelings of helplessness, frustration, and guilt may surface. If the trauma resulted from a man-made error, anger is prominent.

The staff members treating the injured survivors of trauma likewise are recipients of the highly charged emotions of the grief reaction. The injured's initial shock is instinctively countered in the helper by addressing all the physical needs of the patient. The patient's anger is often directed towards those nearest and it is the helper who may experience guilt, indignation and irritation in response to this anger. Staff feelings of hopelessness, guilt, frustration, and helplessness may represent the dysphoria that the victim is experiencing especially if the staff in some way has identified with the victim.

The training of those involved in caring for the trauma victims should prepare them to deal with the emotional reactions [23]. Certain themes occur within helpers with regularity: (1) awareness of their own mortality; (2) awareness of the pain of possibly losing their own family members and friends; (3) sense of relief for not dying nor losing family members this is often followed by guilty feelings, and (4) sense of isolation, that no one understands what they experienced unless they had also gone through it [1, 38].

These themes can be discussed during training and also during staff

meetings or debriefing sessions following disasters. Angry hostile feelings can be aired during staff meetings and the staff can be helped to
recognize that they may simply be reflective of the patient's feelings.
The helpers can be encouraged to discuss their own feelings, painful
memories, and reactions of family/community. In this way, the grief
reactions of these helpers can also be facilitated to reach an adaptive
conclusion.

Grief in Civil Disasters: Special Considerations

The emotional consequences following massive trauma, i.e. disasters, seem to surpass the sum of the individual reactions [see also the
article by *Silverman,* this vol.]. This, in part, is due to unique characteristics of disasters: (1) they are usually sudden an unexpected; (2) the
nature of the disaster is often surreal and awe-inspiring; (3) the large
numbers of deaths are often in the young and previously healthy, and
(4) usually they result in much disfigurement leading to difficulty identifying victims and subsequent uncertainty for the survivors [38]. Survivors of disasters are plunged into simultaneously grieving family
members, friends, and tremendous changes in their environment. Gone
are their homes, foundations for security, nurturing, and sources of
familiarity [39]. Old bonds of kinship and neighborhood are destroyed
[40]. At the time of enormous losses they are faced with relocation and
forced to adjust to new and strange surroundings. One survivor of the
Buffalo Creek flood so graphically stated, 'the flood receded, but the
level of trauma did not: rather, it kept rising, although at a slower pace'
[39].

The focus of the remainder of this paper will be on civil disasters.
Military disaster differ from these mainly by the fact that the military
personnel have undergone a long period of training and preparation for
the actual disaster [22]. It is beyond the intent of this chapter to review
military disasters; however, civil disasters will be reviewed, the grief
reactions initiated by them will be outlined, and guidelines for intervention will be stated.

All of the following civil disasters have been well-chronicled and
it is from these records that generalities of the grief response following
disasters can be drawn.

(1) On the night of November 28, 1942, a fire started in the

basement cocktail lounge of the Coconut Grove nightclub. The club was packed with a Saturday night crowd, the fire spread rapidly, and eventually 491 people lost their lives. Many of the victims and those who subsequently survived were treated at the Massachusetts General Hospital and the Boston City Hospital where neuropsychiatric evaluation and treatment was instituted early [12, 14, 18, 19].

(2) On July 25, 1956, the Swedish liner *Stockholm* rammed into the luxury liner *Andrea Doria*. The fate of the Andrea Doria is well known and has been immortalized in story, song, and film. Less known, the immediate reactions of the survivors have been preserved by two vacationing psychiatrists who were aboard the European-bound liner *Ile de France,* the liner involved in rescuing the survivors of the sinking liner [41].

(3) A massive earthquake hit Skoplje, a city of 200,000 in Yugoslavia on July 26, 1963. Four-fifths of the homes were destroyed, 3,300 people were injured, and 1,070 perished. The Institute of Mental Health in Belgrade sent a psychiatric team consisting of 2 psychiatrists, 1 social worker, and 2 nurses immediately to the disaster site. They arrived within 1 day of the earthquake and remained 5 days [42].

(4) A slag waste dam on the Buffalo Creek Valley in West Virginia collapsed on February 26, 1972, and sent a tidal wave of black sludge down the valley. The homeless numbered 4,000 and 125 were killed. As the survivors initiated litigation, a team of psychiatrists evaluated them fully [39, 40, 43–45].

(5) The Granville Train Disaster resulted January 18, 1977, when a commuter train outside of Sydney, Australia, derailed, hit a bridge, and the bridge collapsed on the train cars. Eighty-three people lost their lives and an equal number were injured. A preventative bereavement intervention program was initiated within the first day of the accident [1, 9, 28, 38].

Four distinct stages of disasters have been described: (1) pre-impact stage (threat); (2) warning stage; (3) impact stage, and (4) post-impact stage (rescue and recovery) [22, 23, 39, 41, 42, 46, 47].

Disasters differ in respect to whether the pre-impact and warning stages exist and if so, their duration. Some disasters are completely without warning while others are well anticipated. The duration of impact and the possible nature of the rescue operations are two other variables which may affect the subsequent reactions [22].

The *pre-impact stage* begins when the probability of a disaster has been announced. This anxiety producing state is greeted by defenses to decrease the anxiety. The result is a successful usage of denial manifested by feelings of personal invulnerability, underactivity or expressions of fatalism [22, 23, 46, 47].

The *warning stage* is that period of imminent danger. The underactivity is replaced by overactivity especially in respect to information gathering. Denial, during this stage, is still the major effective defensive mechanism [46, 47].

The sense of personal invulnerability dramatically changes to feelings of vulnerability and centrality during the *impact stage*. As in the shock phase of individual bereavement, this phase is characterized by a sense of unreality with stunned, dazed, and apathetic behaviors. The lack of expressed affect is quite dramatic even in the presence of obvious injury and emotional trauma [22]. Fifteen to twenty-five percent of survivors can be considered active, efficient helpers during this stage with 20% helpless and unable to even follow directions [23, 42]. The majority are suggestible, docile, unable to make decisions and tend to herd together expressing fears of abandonment, being lost, or separated from their family.

The Andrea Doria survivors behaved as if sedated immediately post-impact [41]. When sedatives were prescribed by the rescuers, very low doses were required to obtain the needed effect. The psychomotor retardation, flat affect, and somnolence were gradually replaced as the sense of unreality waned. Their awareness cleared and they exhibited a great need to tell their story, over and over again, in identical detail to anyone who would listen. Many expressed anger and faulted the crew. There was very little panic and the only psychiatric morbidity occurred in children separated from parents.

As the *post-impact stage* progresses more and more of the survivors are able to participate in and help with the recovery. A sense of euphoria and elation may oscillate with sadness, guilt, helplessness, hopelessness, and despair as the reality of the trauma is appreciated. If human error was involved, anger retaliation, rage, and anxiety may dominate the scene.

The rescue team at Skoplje noted five reactions during this post-earthquake period:

(1) Mild stupor – this sluggishness and apathy was thought to be protective by filtering out incoming stimuli. The stupor was contagious and spread even to the rescue teams.

(2) Escape behavior – often following the after shocks people would spring up ready to flee.

(3) Acute grief – this peaked on the second and third days following the earthquake. Dreams and nightmares were common by night and talking about the catastrophe dominated daytime activities. Children seemed to work through in play what adults would through talking, games of burial and earthquakes were common (this was also seen in children surviving the Buffalo Creek flood).

(4) Superstitious rumors – these spread widely and usually consisted of the theme that the people of Skoplje had lived too well and were now being punished.

(5) Psychosis/panic – very rare [42].

Anxiety, sleep disturbances with nightmares, despair and phobias of water, wind, and rain were common in survivors of the Buffalo Creek flood. Two years following the disaster, 90% of the children had problems with adjustments and development [43]. The post-impact stage of this disaster was heavily influenced by the destruction and subsequent relocation of most the survivors. Possessions, mementoes, and feelings of community were lost. Depressive symptoms and a demoralized state followed in many survivors. With loss of the community, much activity lost direction and purpose. Alcohol and drug usage rose and delinquency among the young became an increasing problem [40].

What guidelines can be established for managing these emotional reactions following disasters? It is clear from the Coconut Groove fire, Skoplje earthquake, and Granville train disaster that the coordinated efforts of diversified agencies and individuals are required. In the pre-impact stage, the community awareness needs to be realistically elevated, positive leadership established, and a relief plan formulated [23, 47]. A good example of this quest for preparedness occurred on May 9, 1967, in Hartford, Conn. To evaluate the performance of a number of agencies, a boiler explosion was simulated [48]. This exercise disclosed numerous problems (victims were inappropriately transported, no clear authority was established at the disaster site, and no one person stayed with the victims to offer comfort and reassurance) which were addressed in future plans for disaster relief.

All disasters cannot be prepared for, nor can all the potential sequellae be anticipated; however, the establishment of relief agencies will help should the disaster occur. *Raphael's* intervention program following the rail disaster is an excellent model of such a coordinated effort [28, 38]. The components of her program organized the labor under these broader headings: (1) counseling; (2) coordination (including public information), and (3) consultation (including education and debriefing).

The counseling team consisted of a group of psychiatrists, social workers with skills in disasters and bereavement, and clergy. This group was stationed at the morgue and was first in contact with the relatives of victims. They primarily offered supportive care and encouraged ventilation of emotions before and during the process of body identification. The additional task of this group was to collect data on survivors to assess relative risk and pass this along to the coordination team. As the counseling team is addressing the needs of the relatives, on-site care is directed at meeting the immediate medical needs of the injured. Rest, warmth, and warm fluids need to be provided to the survivors [14, 23]. Continuity for the excited, confused, and bewildered should be provided [46]. The overly active and agitated should be quickly removed and may need mild sedation [23]. It should be emphasized that by addressing and meeting the medical needs, many of the emotional needs are also met.

The coordination efforts centralized all the information on those affected, assessed their needs, and organized the various agencies involved in relief work. Via the radio, newspapers and television media the community was educated on the effects of the disaster, a survivor list was published, and the public was informed of services available and methods of contact.

The final aspect of their relief program involved consultation. A team of mental health counselors experienced in managing bereavement was gathered to supervise and advise those workers directly servicing the affected families. This work included the debriefing 'grief-work' of the helpers to assist their disengaging from the disaster. It was one final conclusion of *Raphael* that more time and effort should have been expended in this area to help the workers ventilate their feelings and concerns. The consultation team also educated school officials in what to expect in children of victims and what agencies were available for help. This work clearly established the need and the role of the mental health worker in the post disaster period.

Conclusion

Since trauma invariably results in losses at numerous levels, management of the trauma victim involves knowledge of the normal response to losses, the grief reaction. The trauma victim can be monitored to insure and facilitate normal progression of grief. Families of victims similarly require support, education, and may require referral for therapy during the bereavement period. Grief reactions are protective and result in the individual finally being able to give up the ties to the lost object and move forward with their own life forming new relationships. Facilitation of this should be a goal of the comprehensive management of trauma victims.

References

1   Raphael, B.; Singh, B.; Bradbury, L.: Disaster: the helper's perspective. Med. J. Aust. *ii:* 445–447 (1980).

2   Brown, J.T.; Stoudemire, A.: Normal and pathological grief. J. Am. med. Ass. *250:* 378–382 (1983).

3   Viederman, M.; Perry, S.: Use of a psychodynamic life narrative in the treatment of depression in the physically ill. Gen. Hosp. Psychiat. *3:* 177–185 (1980).

4   Hamburg, D.; Hamburg, B.; DeGoza, S.: Adaptive problems and mechanisms in severely burned patients. Psychiatry *16:* 1–20 (1953).

5   Bracken, M.; Shepard, M.: Coping and adaptation following acute spinal cord injury. A theoretical analysis. Paraplegia *18:* 75–85 (1980).

6   Mueller, A.; Thompson, C.: Psychological aspects of the problem in spinal cord injuries. Occup. Ther. Rehab. *29:* 86–95 (1950).

7   Weller, D.; Miller, P.: Emotional reactions of patient, family, and staff in acute-care period of spinal cord injury. Part I. Soc. Work Hlth. Care *2:* 369–377 (1977).

8   Adams, J.; Lindemann, E.: Coping with long-term disability; in Coelho, Hamburg, Adams, Coping and adaptation, pp. 127–138 (Basic Books, New York 1974).

9   Raphael, B.: The Granville train disaster. Psychological needs and their management. Med. J. Aust. *i:* 303–305 (1977).

10   Mueller, A.: Psychological factors in rehabilitation of paraplegic patients. Archs phys. med. Rehabil. *43:* 151–159 (1962).

11   Nagler, B.: Psychiatric aspects of cord injury. Am. J. Psychiat. *107:* 49–55 (1950).

12   Adler, A.: Neuropsychiatric complications in victims of Boston's Coconut Grove disaster. J. Am. med. Ass. *123:* 1098–1101 (1943).

13   Thorn, D.; Salzen, C., von.; Fromme, A.: Psychological aspects of the paraplegic patient. Med. Clins N. Am. *30:* 473 (1946).

14   Cobbs, S.; Lindemann, E.: Coconut Grove burns: neuropsychiatric observations. Ann. Surg. *117:* 814–824 (1943).

15 Wittkower, E.; Gingras, G.; Mesgler, L.; Wigdor, B.; Lepine, A.: Combined psycho-social study of spinal cord lesions. Can. med. Ass. J. *71:* 109–115 (1954).
16 Weller, D.; Miller, P.: Emotional reactions of patient, family, and staff in acute-case period of spinal cord injury. Part II. Soc. Work Hlth. Care *3:* 7–17 (1977).
17 Segall, A.: Sociocultural variation in sick role behavioral expectations. Soc. Sci. Med. *10:* 47–51 (1976).
18 Faxon, N.: Coconut Grove burns: the problems of the hospital administration. Ann. Surg. *117:* 803–813 (1943).
19 Lindemann, E.: Symptomatology and management of acute grief. Ann. J. Psychiat. *101:* 141–148 (1944).
20 Raphael, B.: The Presentation and management of bereavement. Med. J. Aust. *ii:* 909–911 (1975).
21 Parkes, C.: The first year of bereavement. Psychiatry *33:* 444–467 (1970).
22 Engel, G.: Psychological responses to major environmental stress. Grief and mourn-ing; danger, disaster, and deprivation; in Engel, Psychological development in health and disease, pp. 272–287 (Saunders, Philadelphia 1962).
23 Avery, T.: Psychological reactions and other problems in civil disasters. N.Z. med. J. *94:* 348–349 (1981).
24 Clayton, P.; Desmarias, L.; Winokur, G.: A study of normal bereavement. Am. J. Psychiat. *125:* 168–178 (1968).
25 Raphael, B.: Preventative intervention with the recently bereaved. Archs gen. Psychiat. *34:* 1450–1454 (1977).
26 Raphael, B.: The management of pathological grief. Aust. N.Z. J. Psychiat. *9:* 173–180 (1975).
27 Zisook, S.; Devaul, R.; Click, M.: Measuring symptoms of grief and bereavement. Am. J. Psychiat. *139:* 1490–1593 (1982).
28 Singh, B.; Raphael, B.: Post disaster morbidity of the bereaved. J. nerv. ment. Dis. *169:* 203–212 (1981).
29 Maddison, D.; Walker, W.: Factors affecting the outcome of conjugal bereavement. Br. J. Psychiat. *113:* 1057–1067 (1967).
30 Parkes, C.: Determination of outcome following bereavement. Proc. R. Soc. Med. *64:* 279 (1971).
31 Clayton, P.: Mortality and morbidity in the first year of widowhood. Archs gen. Psychiat. *30:* 747–750 (1974).
32 Clayton, P.: The sequellae and nonsequellae of conjugal bereavement. Am. J. Psychiat. *136:* 1530–1534 (1979).
33 Jacobs, S.; Ostfled, A.: An epidemiological review of the mortality of bereavement. Psychosom. Med. *39:* 344–357 (1977).
34 Parkes, C.; Benjamin, B.; Fitzgerald, R.: Br. med. J. *i:* 740–743 (1969).
35 Rees, W.; Lutkin, S.: Mortality of bereavement. Br. med. J. *i:* 13–16 (1967).
36 Bornstein, P.; Clayton, P.; Halikas, J.; Maurice, W.; Robins, E.: The depression of widowhood after thirteen months. Br. med. J. *122:* 561–566 (1973).
37 Parkes, C.; Brown, R.: Health after bereavement. Psychosom. Med. *34:* 449–461 (1972).
38 Raphael, B.: A primary prevention action programme. Psychiatric involvement following a major rail disaster. Omega *10:* 211–225 (1979/80).
39 Rangell, C.: Discussion of the Buffalo Creek disaster. The course of psychic trauma. Am. J. Psychiat. *133:* 313–316 (1976).

40 Erikson, K.: Loss of commuality at Buffalo Creek. Am. J. Psychiat. *133:* 302–305 (1976).

41 Friedmann, P.; Linn, L.: Some psychiatric notes on the Andrea Doria disaster. Am. J. Psychiat. *114:* 426–432 (1957).

42 Popovic, M.; Petrovic, D.: After the earthquake. Lancet *ii:* 1169–1171 (1964).

43 Titchener, J.; Kapp, F.: Family and character change at Buffalo Creek. Am. J. Psychiat. *133:* 295–299 (1976).

44 Stern, G.: From chaos to responsibility. Am. J. Psychiat. *133:* 300–301 (1976).

45 Newman, C.: Children of disaster. Clinical observations at Buffalo Creek. Am. J. Psychiat. *133:* 306–312 (1976).

46 Kinston, W.; Rosser, R.: Disaster. Effects on mental and physical state. J. psychosom. Res. *18:* 437–456 (1974).

47 Glass, J.: Psychological aspects of disaster. J. Am. med. Ass. *171:* 222–225 (1959).

48 Menczer, F.: The Hartford disaster exercise. New Engl. J. Med. *278:* 822–824 (1968).

J. Trig Brown, MD, Division of General Internal Medicine, Duke University Medical Center, Durham, NC 27710 (USA)

Adv. psychosom. Med., vol. 16, pp. 115–140 (Karger, Basel 1986)

Post-Traumatic Stress Disorder

Joel J. Silverman

Consultation-Liaison Psychiatry, Medical College of Virginia, Richmond, Va.,
USA

Introduction and Definitions

Physical and emotional sequelae of traumatic events are brought
to the attention of the public and scientific community on a regular
basis. The consequences of both individual injury and military and
civilian disasters are of increasing importance in psychiatric practice.
This review of post-traumatic stress disorder (PTSD) will begin with
definition and description. Relative risk factors and studies describing
the effects of the syndrome over time will be discussed as well as
examples of physiologic research and treatment issues. Thoughts about
legal intervention and issues for future research will be presented.

PTSD is a psychiatric syndrome which arises in some individuals
following a traumatic stress. Stress is defined as a 'strain, pressure or
tension' [1]. This tension is a 'specific form of disturbance in the
person-environment relationship which initiates psychological and
physiologic responses to facilitate adaptation' [2]. Stressors can be a
combination of physical, psychological, and sociocultural events. Typically, with severe stress, the person is confronted by a harm, threat, or
challenge that cannot be routinely managed and yet must be dealt with
successfully if well-being is to be maintained or enhanced [2]. The ways
in which the stressors affect the recipient's cognitive and physiologic
processes, both consciously and unconsciously, are important. Individuals vary in their ability to perceive dangerous stimuli. They vary
in their assessment of the degree of dangerousness embodied in a given
stimulus and they vary in their response capacity. An experience that
is devastating for one person may have a less severe impact on another,

although literature and lore suggest that there is a stress level which will greatly harm almost anyone.

Certainly, there are usual daily stresses in the lives of adults and children. Typical examples include the pressures of work and school, meeting financial obligations, disagreements with others, the pressures to achieve, and losses of money, prestige, health and loved ones. In order to measure the impact of these daily stresses *Holmes and Rahe* [3] developed a Social Readjustment Scale of desirable and undesirable life events. Changes in these life events have been related to changes in physical and mental health [4]. Most previously healthy human beings respond to these life pressures with mild adjustment or self-limiting grief reactions, but usually without chronic debilitating disease or major ongoing inadequacy of ego function.

Unfortunately, there are catastrophic stresses which are not usually encountered in daily life. These include fires, floods, hostage situations, kidnappings, chemical intoxications, concentration camp and war experiences [5]. These experiences usually embody a stress which overwhelms the individual, threatens or suspends his sense of control, and which contains significant potential for creating many kinds of loss.

People have probably always experienced PTSD. Formal conceptualization of the syndrome began in the 1800s with *Oppenheim* who felt that post-traumatic reactions came from a trauma-induced change in the electrical activity of nerves. This biologic perspective was soon followed by Charcots' explanation that emotional trauma created a negative psychological reaction which could be cured through hypnosis [5]. *Freud* differentiated anxiety from fear, seeing the former as a response to an internal, unconscious threat and the latter a response to external danger. He postulated defense mechanisms as unconscious constructs which protect the organism from excessive stress. He saw anxiety surfacing when repression failed and clearly identified the presence of symptons of autonomic nervous system arousal. Students of *Freud* popularized the post-traumatic phenomenon of 'shell shock' in World War I, and *Freud* [6] wrote of the benefits of using the 'cathartic' method for treating this disorder. Little was known about the underlying physiologic mechanisms until 1936 when *Selye* [7] described the pituitary-adrenal-cortical response to experimental stress which provided physiologic glimpses into the way that stress affects bodily function. *Selye's* [7] general adaptation syndrome described in the 1950s, detailed the characteristic responses to a major threat as alarm, resistance, and ultimately exhaustion. Interest in the interaction of the effects of stress and psychophysiologic functioning increased again as psychiatrists diagnosed soldiers in World War II suffering from 'combat fatigue' or 'battle stress' [8]. Stress in the form of malnutrition, torture, massive family losses, and other psychological hazards of the Nazi concentration camps were also evaluated [9]. These studies, some of which will be discussed below, have even been extended to evaluate the children of holocaust survivors.

Research has also been conducted in nonmilitary populations. In 1941, *Lindemann* [10] studied survivors of the Coconut Grove fire and their relatives. This work was one of the early evaluations of stress syndrome following a civilian disaster, and described a format for grief resolution therapy which ultimately became the basis of many crisis intervention techniques. As one result of military and civilian PTSD evaluations, the term 'gross stress reaction' was included in the 1952 psychiatric diagnostic system, DSM-I, where it was defined as a reversible and transient response to stress. This diagnosis was removed from the DSM-II, only to be returned in significantly modified form in the DSM-III.

The third edition of the Diagnostic and Statistical Manual of the American Psychiatric Association [11] defines acute PTSD (table I) as the 'development of characteristic symptoms following a psychologically traumatic event that is usually outside the range of human experience'. This disorder can occur at any age, and impairment may vary from mild to severe. Individuals repeatedly re-experience the trauma in an intrusive manner and respond to it with psychological numbing or reduced involvement in the external world. Autonomic arousal, often including insomnia, hyper-alertness, and exaggerated startle response, is often chronically present, and patients often experience bursts of anxiety and/or a chronically elevated level of tension. Memory disorder is common, as is avoidance of activities that arouse recollection of the traumatic event. The individual usually vacillates between unpleasant, frightening, intrusive feelings and thoughts reminiscent of the event, and a reactive, powerful tendency to withdraw psychosocially and avoid anything related to the event. This avoidance often generalizes to include phobias, and social and occupational withdrawal.

Acute PTSD has its onset within 6 months of the trauma and lasts less than 6 months. Chronic PTSD lasts 6 months or longer, while the delayed PTSD has its onset at least 6 months after the traumatic event.

Table I. Diagnostic criteria for PTSD

A	Existence of a recognizable stressor that would evoke significant symptoms of distress in almost everyone.
B	Reexperiencing of the trauma as evidenced by at least one of the following

    1 Recurrent and intrusive recollections of the event
    2 Recurrent dreams of the event
    3 Sudden acting or feeling as if the traumatic even were reoccurring, because of an association with an environment or ideational stimulus

C   Numbing of responsiveness to or reduced involvement with the external world, beginning some time after the trauma, as shown by at least one of the following

    1 Markedly diminished interest in one or more significant activities
    2 Feeling of detachment or estrangement from others
    3 Constricted affect

D   At least two of the following symptoms that were not present before the trauma

    1 Hyperalertness or exaggerated starle response
    2 Sleep disturbance
    3 Guilt about surviving when other have not, or about behavior required for survival
    4 Memory impairment or trouble concentrating
    5 Avoidance of activities that arouse recollection of the traumatic event
    6 Intensification of symptoms by exposure to events that symbolize or resemble the traumatic event

This delayed onset, seen frequently in concentration camp survivors and others, is often frighteningly unexpected and seemingly illogical [12]. There is little literature which describes the relative severity and long-term course of these various categories of PTSD.

Diagnostically, PTSD may be confused with an adjustment disorder though in adjustment disorders 'the stressor is usually less severe and within the range of common experience' [11]. Further, the characteristic re-experiencing of the trauma is not routinely seen in adjustment disorders. Patients with PTSD often have accompanying depressive and anxiety disorders which should be additionally diagnosed. Occasionally, severe flashback reactions may be misdiagnosed as schizophrenic behavior. Compensation neurosis may be confused with PTSD. In the former, symptoms are under the subjective control of the patient and have been created based on the patient's conviction that he deserves compensation. PTSD symptoms tend to be unaffected by the presence or absence of compensation [5].

In summary, there is a long history recognizing psychological and psychophysiological responses to severe emotional trauma. Modern diagnostic criteria will improve clinical evaluation and will foster important research studies. One of the most important research problems is determining relative risk factors.

Who Is at Risk?

The risk of developing PTSD appears to be variable and the identification of specific factors which influence risk is difficult. Important interactions do exist between the specific environmental stress and the particular victim. Pre-existing emotional disorder influences both the patient's reaction to the traumatic stress and the long range outcome [13, 14]. *Andreasen* et al. [15] documented increased risk for PTSD in patients with a past history of psychiatric treatment. There is some evidence that the young and elderly are at greater risk, as are those who are single, divorced, or widowed [5]. Unfortunately, specific scientific evidence clarifying the role of personality and past psychiatric illness is limited. There is little evidence that clinicians can predict who will or will not decompensate from a specific stress [16].

The literature documents that many previously healthy individuals experience PTSD after a trauma. About 30% of those who are burned [5], at least one-quarter of Vietnam combat veterans [5], 80% of those involved in the Buffalo Creek Flood [17], most of those involved in the partial collapse of the Kansas City Hyatt House [18], and most children buried in the Chow Chilla bus [19], experienced symptoms of post-traumatic stress disorder. Unfortunately, not all of these studies utilized the same diagnostic criteria, the periods of follow-up were variable, and the patient's prior health status was usually determined retrospectively based upon self report.

The study of *Green* et al. [20] of a catastrophic night club fire in 1977 documents that 60% of the variance in determining the vulnerability to post-traumatic stress comes from factors associated with the traumatic experience itself. PTSD was greater in individuals whose lives were at greater risk, and in those who experienced more bereavement and longer trauma exposure. In situations where the community and its social services were greatly disordered, the likelihood of PTSD increased. It is necessary to replicate this work which suggests that preexisting factors are not the major determinants of susceptibility to developing PTSD. Further work is necessary to clarify the role of personality, coping styles, social support, and prior illness on the risks of developing PTSD and upon the type, severity or length of the syndrome.

The effect of PTSD on families is another important yet insufficiently explored area. Some information is available from the study of the Buffalo Creek flood where the families were also victims directly involved in the trauma [21]. These families were significantly affected with increased alcohol consumption, cigarette smoking, use of prescription drugs, and an increase in juvenile delinquency in the years following the trauma. School-age children seemed to be more severely impaired than younger children, and there was evidence that impairment in children was related to emotional impairment in their parents and disruption of their home. The degree of post-traumatic psychological impairment of one spouse affected the other.

A number of studies have looked at the role of families in post-traumatic adjustment. In studies of long-term adjustment and adaptation to severe burns in adults, *Andreaseon and Norris* [22] pointed out that adults often have difficulty reintegrating into their families after a prolonged hospitalization. The resumption of functioning within the family was seen as 'the strongest single factor in ...(the)... recovery of a sense of continuity and sameness'. The spouses of burn patients remained loyal and demonstrated love and reassurance, but some patients experienced troubling physical withdrawal from their spouses. Wilkinson used a questionnaire to evaluate family support following the Hyatt-Regency skywalk collapse. Eighty percent of involved respondents felt that their family members were 'concerned and supportive' while 20% did not [18].

The holocaust is an extreme but instructive example of the effects of traumatic stress on the family. Important contributions to this literature have been made by children of survivors who have become professionals and have chosen this area to study. Concentration camp survivors themselves experience chronic anxiety and obsessional rumination about their traumatic experiences. Many have great difficulty enjoying life or trusting, and often experience chronic hopelessness and emptiness [23]. Stimuli that disrupt denial and evoke old memories, often elicit reactions of shame or aggression [12]. Survivor guilt and paranoia with hypochondriacal features are also often present. These parental characteristics affect the children. *Russell* [23] described family therapy with 36 survivor families. He conceptualized that ' the adolescent identified patient was the family symptom bearer, expressing the family's pain...' These youngsters experienced academic failure, behavior disorder, depression, problems with identity and sexual functioning, and pyschosomatic complaints. They experienced major guilt about bringing any further suffering to their parents. Even mild rebellion was therefore difficult. Siegel hypothesized that chronic severe parental deprivation reappears in the later parent-child relationships and affects the development of the youngster [24]. *Klein* noted that concentration camp survivors reduced 'grief and separation anxiety' by entering into inadequate marriages prematurely [25]. A number of researchers suggest that the children of survivors feel an excessive pressure to provide meaning for the lives of their parents [12, 26]. The children may serve as 'restitutive lost objects' symbolically replacing relatives lost in camps. These children are at risk of reawakening painful memories and reactions from their parents [12]. *Trossman* [27] described depression and guilt in survivors' children and saw these symptoms as a response to parental overprotectiveness. *Eaton* et al. [28] studied randomly selected heads of Jewish households in Montreal. Seventy percent completed a 1-hour questionnaire including several hundred questions and the Langner Measure of Mental Health. 135 of the 657 respondents were holocaust survivors though not all had been in concentration camps. The authors found that survivors had significantly more psychiatric symptoms than controls though long-term effects on physical health seemed slight. Unfortunately there was no control for death rates in the two populations.

In summary, best evidence suggests that sufficient trauma will create post-traumatic stress disorder in almost anyone. The nature and degree of trauma seem to be more powerful predictors of PTSD symptomatology than preexisting personality. Children of victims suffer from psychopathology which is related to the traumatic experiences of their parents. Families of victims are at risk for suffering, though little is known about the specifics of the positive and negative interactions of victim and family. Future research should expand evaluation of the role of pre-existing factors upon outcome and should explore variables like social support and stress innoculation (gradual exposure to stress) which may be protective or therapeutic.

Intermediate and Long-Range Outcome Studies

A number of studies provide descriptive follow-up of PTSD patients. A few of long-term follow-up studies evaluated stress reactions in World War II combat and noncombat veterans. *Archibald and Tuddenham* [29] studied 62 World War II veterans who still had gross stress reactions 20 years after the war. These veterans were studied using a questionnaire and the MMPI and were compared to a group of noncombat veterans with psychiatric complaints and to combat veterans who were psychiatrically well. Twenty years after the war, the combat fatigue group had more 'combat dreams, momentary blackouts, sweating of hands or feet, diarrhea, excessive jumpiness, severe headaches... dizziness, depression, easily fatigued, excessive smoking and heart pounding.' New cases of the delayed type increased with time. Six percent of the sample had presented at the clinic by 1950; between 1951 and 1960, 60% of the sample presented; and the last 32% presented between 1961 and 1964. Patients confirmed that the frequency of their symptoms increased over time since the combat experience. The authors were also impressed that these men were loners who avoided communication and emotions.

Cognition and affect play important roles in the long-term experience of PTSD, *Sifneos* [30] described alexithymia, the inability to express or name emotions, as an important characteristic of individuals with psychosomatic illness. The inability to verbally express emotion is postulated to be related to increased emotional expression through psychophysiologic symptomatology. Though the etiology of alexithymia is unknown, it is postulated that inadequate brain development and early learning may be influential. In 1983, *Shipko* et al. [31] measured alexthymia in 23 Vietnam combat veterans who met DSM-III criteria for PTSD. Nine individuals (41%) scored 50 or below on the Schaling-Sifnoes alexithymia scale, five times the expected frequency of alexithymia in normative data. Even though these individuals were tested 10–15 years after combat stress, they continued to note lack of emotion following important events such as the death of a parent or the birth of a child. Unfortunately, the authors did not evaluate non-PTSD combatants as controls and the precombat alexithymia status of these subjects was unknown. It may be that there is a primary alexithymia which begins early in life and a secondary syndrome which follows trauma. This study should be replicated, since it may offer information about another link between stress and its psychophysiologic antecedents and sequelae.

In 1963, *Leopold and Dillon* published a 3½- to 4½-year follow-up study of 27 seamen who were involved in a tanker-freighter collision in the Delaware River [32]. Nine of the men suffered mild concussion and 14 had abrasions and lacerations. The rest were physically uninjured. Patients were evaluated psychiatrically immediately following the disaster and no systematic psychiatric care was available in the interim. The effects of litigation on outcome were mitigated because compensation is afforded to seamen by statue without litigation. Ninety percent of the men were 25–50 years old at the time of the accident. Five were high school graduates and most had long service at sea and were familiar with dangerous conditions. Results revealed that pre-existing personal or family background did not predict postdisaster psychopathology. Patients endorsed 'moderate' pretrauma drinking, though there was no quantitative documentation of alcohol intake. Most of the patients had multiple psychological and psychosomatic complaints following the incident, including disorders of mood, sleep disturbance, and gastrointestinal complaints.

At 4½ years follow-up, significant psychological deterioration was noted. Twenty-six of the men received some form of help for psychiatric complaints and 12 had been hospitalized. Ten suffered severe gastrointestinal manifestations. Affective disturbances had more than doubled and there was a marked increase in restlessness, phobia, and sleep disorder. New complaints included feelings of isolation, a perception of being watched, and a sense of hostility. Unfortunately, no follow-up measures of alcohol use were included. At follow-up, well over half of the patients complained of continuous and sometimes disabling headache. It is further worth noting the uncontrolled observation that 4 of the 34 never returned to work at sea, 12 briefly returned and then gave up this occupation, and 6 worked only sporadically. A greater degree of psychological deterioration was noted in the subjects who were older at the initial trauma. The authors concluded that very significant debility was evident in 70% of this population at follow-up.

A more recent report evaluated the aftermath of a maritime collision between the USS Belknap and the USS Kennedy [33]. Forty-six of the Belknap's crew were injured and 8 died. The authors compared medical records before and after the tragedy for 25 officers and 311 crew and compared these with medical records from the same time period of 387 officers and crew of a similar mission without mishap. Precollision personality and psychiatric data were similar for personnel on both ships with the exception that the control crew had more psychiatric hospitalizations. Following the collision, 13 men from the control ship experienced psychiatric hospitalization 'three each for alcoholism, schizophrenia and transient situational disturbance and two each for personality disorder and special symptoms'. Eighteen members of the Belknap received psychiatric hospitalization, 13 for neuroses, 4 with transient situational disturbance, and 1 for alcoholism. None of these men had been previously hospitalized psychiatrically. The difference in the specific type of psychiatric diagnoses for the two crews were highly significant, the Belknap crew mainly suffering from neuroses. Further, more members of the Belknap were medically separated from the service following collision. An additional 35 Belknap sailors were treated for PTSD symptoms in outpatient settings. This study provides reasonable assessment of precollision variables and demonstrates a significant increase in postcollision neuroses.

Another methodologically sound research was conducted by *Glesser* et al. [21] who studied the effect on the Buffalo Creek community of a massive, destructive flood that followed the disruption of a coal waste dam in West Virginia in 1972. Two years after the flood, most survivors remained so debilitated that their symptoms interfered with their daily lives. Only 1 in 6 of the adult victims was considered entirely asymptomatic, and at least 35% were considered to be moderately to severely disturbed even though they had received many brief therapeutic interventions. Thirty percent of subjects evaluated 4–5 years postdisaster continued to suffer significant debilitating symptoms. Families reported a 30% increase in alcohol consumption, 44% more cigarette smoking, and a 52% increase in the use of prescription medications. Juvenile delinquency increased 12%. Over 75% of the Buffalo Creek respondents reported serious problems with sleep more than two years after the flood.

Follow-up studies in traumatized children are limited. In 1976, a school bus in Chowchilla, Calif., was hijacked [19]. Twenty-six children, ages 5–14 years, disappeared for 27 hours and were buried alive in their bus. They dug themselves out and were subsequently evaluated. At the time of initial reporting, it was noted that 'each child suffered post-traumatic emotional sequelae'. A follow-up study published in 1983 documented that 'even though some of the more dramatic manifestations of psychic trauma (exact repetition of dreams and some fears) disappeared over time, a significant trauma continued to exert an influence on the daily life, personality development and future expectations of previously normal children [34]. Every child was found to suffer from a post-traumatic stress syndrome as late as 4–5 years after the incident. In this study, the post-traumatic symptoms of the children differed from those usually seen in adults in that the children did not experience amnesia, psychic numbing or intrusive flashbacks. School performance remained relatively stable. The children did evidence reenactment of the trauma in their play, effects on personality development and difficulty remembering the appropriate time frames of events within the trauma. They did not deny the existance of the trauma. Children also evidenced a reduction of hopefulness about their future. This nonblind, uncontrolled study, concluded that 'children are not more flexible than adults following a pure psychic trauma'.

These studies emphasize the widespead, long-term influence of trauma on psychological and psychophysiologic function in individuals who were apparently normal before the traumatic occurence.

PTSD and Pentaborane Intoxication

This authors' experience with PTSD began in February, 1982, when 3 industrial workers were attempting to detoxify old pentaborane-filled cannisters. Pentaborane (B5H9) is a highly volatile liquid boron hydride which is extremely active reducing substance possessing a high degree of toxicity equal or greater than hydrocyanide [35, 36]. This substance has been widely used in industry as a catalyst in synthetic reactions and is a parent compound in the synthesis of carborane polymers and is a dopant in the manufacture of semiconductors [37]. Pentaborane can be absorbed by inhalation, ingestion, or through the skin. It reacts vigorously with ammonia, organic amines, unsaturated hydrocarbons and various heterocycloamines, and therefore is highly destructive to tissue, especially in the central nervous system. Animal research confirms that boron hydrides selectively react with nervous tissue and probably deplete the central nervous system of monoamine neurotransmitters [38–40].

The industrial workers became acutely ill at the scene and rescue personnel and bystanders were briefly intoxicated. One worker died

Table II. Pentborane evaluation

Medical and personal history	Mental status examination
Physical and neurologic examination	Diagnostic interview schedule
Neuropsychological assessment	Plasma CSF neurotransmitter studies
Electroencephalogram	Antibrain antibodies
CT scan	
Complete blood count	Urinalysis
Dexamethasone suppression test	Serology
Thyroid function	SMA-20
Pulmonary function	B12/folate

with massive central nervous system degeneration. Another worker remained unconscious for months and ultimately sustained major neurologic deficit. The third worker had grand mal seizures, disorientation, agitation and hallucinations but ultimately improved [41].

Our study involved the neuropsychiatric evaluation of the 14 rescue squad personnel and bystanders who were briefly exposed [42]. They were formally evaluated by us in the hospital approximately 4–6 weeks following exposure. Seven men and 7 women with a mean age of 26.3 ± 8 years were studied. Their mean educational level at the time of exposure was 13.7 ± 1.6 years. Three were students, 10 were employed, and 1 was a homemaker. Three were married, 10 single, and 1 was separated. All were in good previous health except 1 patient who was being treated with steroids for Addison's disease and another patient who had a past history of mild asthma. One patient had a reported history of counseling for marital maladjustment 4 years prior to exposure.

Evaluation (table II) included medical and personal histories, physical and neurologic examination, routine blood chemistries, a semistructured mental status examination, psychiatric diagnoses using the fully scripted Diagnostic Interview Schedule [43], neuropsychological assessment, and extensive laboratory evaluation. Patients received electroencephalograms, computerized tomography (CT scan) of the head and blood was collected for monoamine measurements. The first eight individuals underwent lumbar puncture for measurement of cerebrospinal fluid neurotransmitters and antibrain antibodies. A retrospective estimate of initial exposure was constructed based on initial patient reports of proximity and length of exposure to pentaborane.

Table III. Patients experiencing each symptom in the first 36 hours

Symptom/Sign	n	%	Symptom/Sign	n	%
Lightheaded	14	100	Rash	6	43
Confused	13	93	Feel drunk	5	36
No energy	13	93	Waves through head	5	36
Insomnia	13	93	Sick to stomach	5	36
Can't concentrate	12	86	Visual hallucinations	4	29
Nightmares	11	79	Chills or fever	4	29
Tightness in chest	11	79	Can't get breath	4	29
Vision blurred	11	79	Memory loss	3	21
React badly	9	64	Don't feel safe	3	21
Tightness in throat	9	64	Sleeping longer	3	21
Muscle jerks	9	64	Appetite less	3	21
Feel detached	7	50	Appetite more	2	14
Strange taste	7	50	Can't swallow	2	14
Headache	7	50	Walks in sleep	1	7
Numbness	7	50	Vomits	1	7

Initially, following exposure patients experienced lightheadedness, confusion, loss of energy, insomnia, poor concentration, tightness in the chest and visual blurring. These signs and symptoms are noted in table III. More than half experienced bloody nightmares. During the first day patients had conjunctivitis and facial rash. One patient experienced a generalized seizure, 9 had myoclonic jerks, and 3 complained of memory loss while 4 experienced visual hallucinations. As characteristic of pentaborane toxicity, symptoms increased on the day following exposure and ten rescue squad members were admitted to another hospital. Seven of the 10 had positive electroencephlograms which showed bitemporal theta waves compatible with toxic encephalopathy.

Four to 6 weeks after the traumatic exposure, all patients had normal physical and neurologic examinations except the patient with Addisonian hyperpigmentation. Routine laboratory tests, thyroid and pulmonary function tests were normal as were the B-12/folate, anti-brain antibodies, and dexamethasone suppression test. The initial mental status examination and independent questionnaire measures revealed that 50% of the patients met DSM-III criteria for PTSD. In addition, 4 patients with PTSD and 2 patients who did not have PTSD had clinically important depressive symptoms though they did not then meet DSM-III Major Affective Disorder criterion for length of illness. Patients who had a diagnosis of PTSD at 4–6 weeks postexposure had experienced more early symptoms of pentaborane intoxication than those who did not develop PTSD. Patients endorsed recurrent bloody dreams and thoughts of the event, startle responses, hyperalertness, marked diminished interest in one or more significant activities, feelings of detachment from others, and constricted affect. At 4–6 weeks following intoxication, 64% of patients were experiencing lethargy, 57% difficulty concentrating, 57% poor emotional control, 50% continued to have insomnia and 43% reported nightmares. These finding of post-traumatic stress disorder were at marked variance with previous reports of pentaborane intoxication which had failed to reveal any significant continuation of symptoms beyond 2 weeks postexposure.

It is worth noting that measurements of ventricular/brain ratio (VBR), a CT scan finding, for 12 of the pentaborane patients revealed CT scan ratios of $8.08 + .03$ as compared to a control value ($n = 29$) of $3.45 + 2.7$. The difference between these means was statistically significant ($t = 4.39$, $p < 0.001$). One of the fourteen patients refused CT scan and the patient with Addison's disease had the largest ventricular/brain ratio but was excluded from analysis because of the distant possibility that replacement steroids may have affected her VBR. Thirty-eight percent (5 patients) of this sample had VBRs between 1 and 2 SDs above the control group mean and another five patients had VBRs greater than 2 SDs above the control group mean. Evidence suggests that an enlarged VBR is compatible with central nervous system disorder since it is also found in many alcoholics and in some patients with schizophrenia and head injury [44–46]. Further evidence of organic brain damage came from deficits which existed on 5 of 11 neuropsychological tests, including measures of sustained attention, memory and visuospatial problem solving. 36–57% of these patients were impaired on five measures of neuropsychological function [47]. The Hopkins Symptom Checklist revealed significant elevations in the anxiety and obsessive compulsive subscales. Plasma and spinal fluid neurotransmitters were elevated. The 7 patients who were diagnosed as having PTSD were encouraged to receive psychiatric care. Only 2 accepted this recommendation within the first year and a half.

A second evaluation was completed approximately a year and a half after the initial trauma. Results revealed that neuropsychological testing improved and the CT scan VBR remained unchanged. The

Table IV. Psychiatric diagnosis

	Initial	Follow-up
PTSD, acute	7	
PTSD, chronic		4
PTSD, delayed		3
Major affective disorder	6	4
Alcohol abuse		2
Phobia		2
	13 diagnosis	17 diagnosis

mental status examination (table IV) revealed that 4 of the 7 patients with initial PTSD continued to have the disorder at follow-up, therefore meeting criteria for chronic PTSD. An additional 3 previously undiagnosed patients developed delayed reactions and there were four DSM-III diagnoses of major affective disorder, two of alcohol abuse, and two of phobia. In the interim, 2 patients had been suicidal, and 7 patients had dramatic shifts in school performance or experienced major job problems.

In conclusion, a year and a half following the experience of the central nervous system intoxication coupled with the psychological trauma of being acutely exposed to a dangerous, little known substance, patients showed improvement in neuropsychological functioning, stability in CT scan VBR but no overall improvement in the prevalence of psychopathology. These findings of extended debility in this young, previously healthy sample are consistent with findings of other long-term studies which demonstrate ongoing serious pathology. These studies reinforce the need to explore the potential of protective value of early treatment in PTSD.

Physiologic Concomitants of PTSD

The findings of long-term psychological and psychophysiologic symptoms in the pentaborane population and others with PTSD is a clinically expected part of the syndrome. *Pavlov* [48] first explored autonomic responses to experimental trauma in animals and people. This early work was extended to experimental evaluation of post-combat physiologic responses to simulated combat stress by *Dobbs and Wilson* [49] in 1961. These investigators evaluated heart rate, respiration, and alpha EEG waves in combat veterans with uncompensated combat neuroses. Subjects were exposed to taped combat sounds and photostimulation. Although the authors did not fully present specific outcome, there was a 'remarkable similarity of the behavior and physiologic responses of the war neurotics to those produced experimentally in animals through conditioning'. In 1982, *Blanchard* et al. [50] replicated this work. They studied 11 DSM-III diagnosed PTSD Viet Nam veterans, 32–42 years old. Controls were 11 males of approximately the same age who had no Vietnam military experience. Heart rate, blood pressure, peripheral surface temperature, forehead muscle activity, and skin resistance were studied. Subjects were exposed to continuous combat sounds for up to 480 seconds with gradually increasing intensity. Significant increases in heart rate, systolic blood pressure, and forehead EMG were noted in veterans listening to combat sounds. Controls did not change. Discriminate function analysis demonstrated that the best physiologic discriminator was heart rate which correctly discriminated 21 of the 22 subjects. The 1 subject incorrectly classified was receiving haloperidol at assessment. The authors conclude that the veterans showed significantly more physiologic avoidant behavior many years following their Vietnam experience.

Sleep is a physiological parameter which is frequently abnormal in both military and civilian PTSD. Some authors view sleep disorder as the primary cause of the other signs and symptoms of PTSD [51]. Laboratory sleep studies in PTSD have provided conflicting results. One author recommended benzodiazepine treatment for patients with night terror/nightmares, a non-REM, stage 4 sleep event associated with nocturnal motor activity and poor dream recall. This author utilized REM suppressing monoamine oxidase inhibitors for patients with dream anxiety attacks, which are REM events associated with good dream recall [51]. *Burstein* [52], in an uncontrolled study, found a high incidence of sleep disorder in PTSD veterans which responded well to treatment with imipramine (mean dose 260 mg).

Another important psychophysiologic area of research is the animal model of learned helplessness postulated by *Maier and Seligman* [53]. This model is based upon the experimental observation that animals exposed to inescapable aversive conditions, such as pain, loud noise, or cold water, later show difficulty escaping from new aversive situations, difficulty with new learning, and chronic evidence of distress. There is remarkable similarity between the animals' hyperalert and avoident behaviors following experimental stress and clinical PTSD. Further, animals exposed to the learned helplessness pardigm have increased norepinephrine turnover, increased plasma catecholamine levels, reduction in brain norepinephrine, and increased MPHG production [54, 55]. These animal findings are similar to the monoamine elevations in the pentaborane patients. In animal studies of learned helplessness, clonidine, benzodiazepines, tricyclic antidepressants, monoamine oxidase inhibitors have been shown to reduce abnormal behavior [56]. Many of these drugs also have reported clinical utility in humans with PTSD.

There is great potential to expand our understanding of the psychopathophysiology of PTSD. It is possible that acute stress affects neuroendocrine systems in a manner that abnormally maintains a hypervigilant posture and lowers the threshold of arousal. Systematic controlled study of physiologic baselines and responses to treatments is required.

Treatment of PTSD

There is an important literature describing various pharmacological, psychotherapeutic, and behavioral treatments for PTSD. Most studies are short-term and suggest improvement in response to treatment. Weaknesses in these studies include variability in diagnostic criteria, lack of blind assessments, lack of standardization of the therapy, and the realistic problems obtaining appropriate control groups. A review of this literature fails to provide a clear statement about a treatment of choice or even appropriate indication for specific interventions.

Many of the PTSD treatment articles have been associated with combat experiences. Early studies in patients with shellshock recommended prompt treatment in close proximity to the battlefield. An article from the Viet Nam era outlined similar principles for military management of PTSD [57]. Immediacy, brevity were recommended as well as proximity to the combat zone. Therapist and patients were to have high expectations for a hasty return to combat and therapy was to avoid past issues and attend to the 'here and now'. The use of psychopharmacologic agents, especially sedatives, was deemphasized in this report though other military psychiatrists have emphasized the use of short duration high dose antipsychotic therapy to induce 2–3 days of intense sleep. The military hoped that these treatment approaches, coupled with a time limited combat experience for each soldier, breaks for rest and relaxation, and on site presence of mental health support personnel would lower the incidence of psychiatric illness. While some claimed success, much evidence suggests that these interventions were inadequate to address the psychopathology of our soldiers [58].

Lifton [59], discussing PTSD therapy for veterans, recommended the creation of nonanalytic self-help rap groups. He suggested that fear of death underlied the PTSD in many veterans. In addition, these veterans also feared betrayal and abandonment and experienced guilt and grief about their own dehumanization and their dehumanized behavior associated with the need to survive in a war zone [59]. Group therapy was seen as highly valuable since it neutralized resistance, dealt with trust and authority problems, and addressed guilt and the need for camaraderie. Many authors have emphasized the need to explore the extreme denial in PTSD patients which often impedes the processing of appropriate issues [60, 61]. *Ewalt and Crawford* [62], discussing group therapy with Viet Nam veterans, supported a reality orientation, the use of abreaction, and the avoidance of regression. *Rosenheim and Elizur* [63], in discussing the Yom Kippur war, emphasized the need to quickly reestablish precrisis levels of functioning. He felt that the first stage of his group therapy related to the expression and realization of open pain and regression. In this phase, patients became increasingly narcissistic, withdrawn, and dependent upon group support and cohesion. A more realistic perspective was established in the second phase of therapy when patients worked through the reality of their situation and explored questions, such as 'What will people think of me for breaking down under stress?' In the last stage, problem-solving predominated and patients resumed normal functioning having assessed the costs of remaining ill. A healthy separation from the group was then possible.

Individual psychoanalysis and psychotherapy have been reported with mixed results in patients with PTSD. *Terr* [34], working with the children traumatized at Chow Chilla, felt that brief therapy demonstrated little benefit. Horowitz explicated tasks of psychotherapy including (1) decreasing external stress; (2) decreasing oscillation between denial and intrusive thoughts; (3) encouraging expression and control of trauma-related thoughts; (4) working through the meaning of the trauma for the individual; (5) increasing self-image, and (6) improving relationships [64].

A number of authors have emphasized the need to assess countertransference issues [61, 63, 65]. The leader must be able to tolerate the affect of the goup as well as his/her feelings about the trauma. This is particularly difficult when the trauma is so horrible that it awakens revulsion in the leader or has actually touched the leader's life. Lindy pointed out that therapists involved in the early physical resolution of trauma, such as the recovery and identification of bodies may, indeed, be victims themselves and may find it difficult to deal with their feelings about the trauma [67].

A variety of psychopharmacologic agents alone and in combination with psychotherapy have been used in treating PTSD. Benzodiazepines and sedatives generally are seen as having limited effectiveness though narcoanalysis has been used with mixed results since World War II [65]. A number of authors have studied and recommend tricyclic antidepressants [57, 66]. Pentaborane patients with PTSD and depressive symptoms responded well to doxepin at both therapeutic and subtherapeutic plasma levels. *Hogben and Kornfield* provided an interesting report of 5 PTSD patients who were previous treatment failures with antipsychotics, tricyclic antidepressants, and psychotherapy who responded well to a nonblind trial of phenelzine [68]. This medication was felt to enhance psychotherapy and its effect inhibiting REM stage dreams was believed to be particularly beneficial. Low-dose antipsychotics have been recommended for PTSD patients with paranoia, anger, self-destructiveness and flashbacks though no controlled studies have been reported. *Kolb* et al. have written about the use of beta-blockers and the alpha$_2$-receptor blockade of clonidine. These studies are based on the belief that 'persisting conditioned emotional response does exist in the groups of PTSD sufferers' [69]. Propranolol blocks adrenergic response and has been used successfully to treat anxiety and panic. Clonidine has been used to reduce anxiety and narcotic withdrawal. In animal studies, it blocks alpha$_2$-receptors in the norepinephrine rich locus ceruleus which is believed to affect fear responses. The use of these

agents in PTSD appears promising though additional blind controlled
studies are required. Case reports exist describing a variety of other
therapies, including systematic desensitization, hypnosis, and
implosion therapy.

There is a major need for long-term, systematic, well-controlled
treatment studies with blind standardized assessment. Group psychotherapy and tricyclics have been used most extensively to treat PTSD.
MAOIs, beta- and alpha$_2$-blockers are promising as therapeutic agents.
Few studies have explored the effect of early treatment upon outcome.

Legal Problems

There are many important legal issues associated with PTSD,
including dealing with crimes committed by PTSD patients and suits
to recover damages associated with PTSD. The psychiatrist can function in a variety of important capacities. A veteran in Rockville, Md.,
in 1979 held bank patrons hostage for over 6 hours [70]. The accused
claimed that he was reliving a war-time event and saw the police as
enemy soldiers and his hostages as allies he was protecting. This veteran
was placed on probation. Thousands of other Viet Nam veterans are
currently incarcerated in this country. The incidence of PTSD in this
group and the relationship of PTSD to their legal difficulty are unknown. The Veterans Administration and the American Psychiatric
Association accept PTSD as a potential defense in certain legal situations.

Another common legal-PTSD situation occurs when patients attempt to recover damages claiming to suffer from post-traumatic stress
disorder. In the pentaborane case, the industrial defendants responded
by denying the validity of PTSD and accusing the patients of malinger-
ing. In contrast to malingerers, these patients used excessive denial and
were reluctant to utilize medical and psychiatric evaluation or care.
This denial of illness and avoidance of medical care has been well
reported in many PTSD studies. On the other hand, there is an anecdotal literature casting doubt upon the validity of post-traumatic syndromes by asserting that they are motivated and sustained by greed and
disappear following the application of financial settlement or the 'green
poultice'. *Breaverman* [71], studying PTSD in Austria where litigation
is not usually necessary to obtain compensation, showed that the

incidence of post-traumatic disorder was unrelated to issues of financial gain in various types of injuries. The study of *Leopold and Dillon* [32] of the seamen involved in the Delaware River disaster revealed a high incidence of long-term post-traumatic stress symptoms and debility, even though the Maritime Compensation Act precluded the necessity of litigation [32]. The investigators of the Buffalo Creek disaster did a pilot study of involved nonlitigants and found a similar incidence of psychiatric disorder in both nonlitigants and litigants [21]. *Kelly* [72] studied head injured patients finding that 84 of 110 returned to work prior to the settlement of claims. Seventy percent of these patients injured in settings where no claim was appropriate or filed, nevertheless experienced post-traumatic stress disorder. *Kelly* felt that return to work was related to proper medical recognition and treatment of PTSD symptoms rather than to the questions of pending compensation.

The task of providing psychiatric testimony remains difficult. Communicating the nature and reality of PTSD to a jury of a lay persons who have not personally experienced it, is indeed challenging. At the time of trial, the PTSD patients often appear physically and emotionally normal and have returned to work. In order to document the diagnosis, a careful, unbiased history of symptoms from the patient and family members is necessary. Discovery of a reasonably consistent, independently presented symptom pattern in many patients similarly traumatized lends credance to the diagnosis. The use of standard Diagnostic Interview Schedule, facilitates objectivity on the part of psychiatrists for both the defense and prosecution. The use of videotape for documenting initial information to be used later in court requires considerable study since the taping may alter patient and physician behavior. The pentaborane patients, like rape victims, found that depositions and testimony were extremely stressful. These legal activities precipitated a reliving of the trauma with its painful memories, feelings, and dreams. Guilt, shame, and embarrassment were reawakened. Helpful defenses of denial, isolation of affect, and avoidance were weakened. The explicit attacks upon the veracity of patient accounts generated rage and resonated with some patient's implicit self-doubt. The psychiatrist has an important role in helping the patient process this distressing material. Attorneys are aware that this distress increases the patient's desire to settle the case and avoid courtroom confrontation.

Future Research

While important strides have been made to improve the systematic study of trauma victims, extensive work remains. Methods and general designs for studying trauma should be developed in advance to be ready for modification and application to specific situations. Studies must incorporate standardized diagnostic criteria. To do this the development of improved, valid, reliable measures of PTSD is a high priority [73]. Use of objective biologic measurements to document stress-related changes will hopefully expand. Scientific methodology should be applied to the comparative study of all therapies to develop a clear idea of which treatment or combination of treatments should be applied in each situation. Research should be expanded to explore the role of personality, prior trauma experience and social support in the vulnerability to trauma, in the natural history of PTSD and in responses to treatment. Research should explore the differential experience of experiencing a trauma as an individual versus the effect of trauma when experienced with others. Exploration of the role of denial and alexithymia could help overcome resistance to treatment. Unfortunately, it is unlikely that the incidence of civilian and military trauma will be reduced. The development of better tools to identify and treat victims is necessary.

References

1   Webster's New Universal Unabridged Dictionary; 2nd ed. (Simon & Schuster, New York 1979).
2   Benner, P.; Roskies, E.; Lazrus, R.: Stress in coping under extreme conditions; in Dimsdale, Survivors, victims, and perpetrators. Essays on the Nazi holocaust, chap. 9 (Hemisphere, Washington 1980).
3   Holmes, T.H.; Rahe, R.: The social readjustment rating scale. J. psychosom. Res. *11:* 213–218 (1967).
4   Braunstein, J.J.: Reactions to stress; in Braunstein, Toister, Medical applications of the behavioral sciences, chap. 7 (Yearbook Medical Publishers, Chicago 1981).
5   Andreason, N.J.C.: Post-traumatic stress disorder; in Kaplan, Friedman, Sadock, Comprehensive textbook of psychiatry, vol. III, pp. 1517–1525 (Williams & Wilkins, New York 1980).
6   Freud, S.: Introduction to psychoanalysis and the war neurosis (1919); in London, Complete psychological works, vol. 17 (Hogarth Press, London 1959).
7   Selye, H.: The stress of life (McGraw-Hill, New York 1956).
8   Grinker, R.R.; Spiegel, J.P.: Men under stress (Blakiston, Philadelphia 1945).

9   Dimsdale, J.E.: Survivors, victims and perpetrators. Essays on the Nazi holocaust (Hemisphere, Washington 1980).

10   Lindemann, E.: Symptomatology and management of acute grief. Am. J. Psychiat. *101:* 141–148 (1944).

11   Diagnostic and statistical manual of mental disorders; 3rd ed. (American Psychiatric Association, Washington 1980).

12   Wilson, A.; Fromm, E.: Aftermath of the concentration camp. The second generation. J. Am. Acad. Psychoanal. *10:* 289–313 (1982).

13   Brill, N.Q.; Beebe, B.W.: A follow-up study of war neuroses. Veterans Administration Medical Monograph (US Government Printing Office, Washington 1955).

14   Hendin, H.; Haas, A.P.: Combat adaptations of Vietnam veterans without post-traumatic stress disorders. Am. J. Psychiat. *141:* 956–960 (1984).

15   Andreasen, N.J.C.; Noyes, R.; Hartford, C.E.: Factors influencing adjustment of burn patients during hospitalization. Psychosom. Med. *34:* 517–525 (1972).

16   Glass, A.J.: Observations upon the epidemiology of mental illness in troops during warfare; in Symposium on preventive and social psychiatry (Walter Reed Army Institute of Research, Washington 1969).

17   Titchener, J.L.; Kapp, F.T.: Family and character changes at Buffalo Creek. Am. J. Psychiat. *133:* 295–299 (1976).

18   Wilkinson, C.B.: Aftermath of a disaster: The collapse of the Hyatt Regency Hotel skywalks. Am. J. Psychiat. *140:* 1134–1139 (1983).

19   Terr, L.C.: Psychic trauma in children. Observations following Chowchilla School bus kidnapping. Am. J. Psychiat. *138:* 14–19 (1981).

20   Green, B.L.; Grace, M.C.; Glesor, G.C.: Identifying survivors at risk: long-term impairment following the Beverly Hills Supper Club fire. J. consult. clin. Psychol. (in press).

21   Gleser, G.C.; Grenn, B.L.; Winget, C.: Prolonged psychosocial effects of disaster. A study of Buffalo Creek (Academic Press, New York 1981).

22   Andreasen, N.J.C.; Norris, A.S.: Long term adjustment in adaptation mechanisms in severely burned adults. J. nerv. ment. Dis. *154:* 352–362 (1982).

23   Russell, A.: Late effects. Influence on the children of the concentration camp survivor; in Dimsdale, Survivors, victims, and perpetrators: essays on the Nazi holocaust, chap. 7 (Hemisphere, Washington 1981).

24   Segal, J.J.; Silver, D.; Rakoff, V.; Ellin, B.: Some second generation effects of survival of the Nazi persecution. Am. J. Orthopsychiat. *43:* 320–327 (1973).

25   Klein, H.: Problems in the psychotherapeutic treatment of Israeli survivors of the Holocaust; in Krystal, Massive psychic trauma (International University Press, New York 1968).

26   Kestenberg, A.: Psychoanalytic contributions to the problems of children survivors from Nazi persecution. Israel Psychiat. Relat. Discipl. *4:* 311–323 (1972).

27   Trossman, B.: Adolescent children of concentration camp survivors. Can. psychiat. Ass. J. *13:* 121–123 (1968).

28   Eaton, W.W.; Sigal, J.J.; Weinfeld, M.: Impairment in Holocaust survivors after 33 years. Data from an unbiased community sample. Am. J. Psychiat. *139:* 773–777 (1982).

29   Archibald, H.C.; Tuddenham, R.D.: Persistent stress reactions after combat. A 20-year follow-up. Archs gen. Psychiat. *12:* 475–481 (1965).

30   Sifneos, P.E.: Clinical observation on patients suffering from a variety of psychoso-
     matic diseases; in Antonelli, Proc. 7th Eur. Conf. Psychosom Res., Rome 1967, pp.
     1–10.

31   Shipko, S.; Alvarez, W.A; Noviello, N.: Towards a teleological model of alexithy-
     mia. Alexithymia and post-traumatic stress disorder. Psychother. Psychosom. *39:*
     122–126 (1983).

32   Leopold, R.L.; Dillon, H.: Psycho-anatomy of disaster. A long-term study of
     post-traumatic neurosis in survivors of a marine explosion. Am. J. Psychiat. *119:*
     913–921 (1963).

33   Hoyberg, A.; McCaughney, B.G.: The traumatic after effects of collision at sea.
     Am. J. Psychiat. *141:* 70–73 (1984).

34   Terr, L.C.: Chowchilla revisited. The effects of psychic trauma four years after a
     school bus kidnapping. Am. J. Psychiat. *141:* 1543–1550 (1983).

35   Mindrum, G.: Pentaborane intoxication. Archs intern. Med. *114:* 364–374 (1964).

36   Roush, G.: The toxicology of the boranes. J. occup. Med. *1:* 32–46 (1959).

37   Hurd, D.T.: An introduction to the chemistry of the hydrides (Wiley, New York
     1952).

38   Merritt, J.H.; Schultz, E.J.; Wykes, A.A.: Effect of decarborane on the norepine-
     phrine content of rat brain. Biochem. Pharmac. *13:* 1364–1366 (1964).

39   Merritt, J.H.; Schultz, E.J.: The effect of decaborane on the biosynthesis and
     metabolism of norepinephrine in the rat brain. Life Sci. *5:* 27–32 (1966).

40   Back, K.C.: Aerospace toxicology. I. Propellant toxicology. Fed. Proc. *29:*
     2000–2005 (1970).

41   Yarborough, B.E.; Garrettson, L.K.; Zolet, D.; Cooper, K.; Kelleher, B.; Healy,
     P.: Severe central nervous system damage and profound acidosis in persons exposed
     to pentaborane. Clin. Toxicol. *7:* 23 (1985).

42   Silverman, J.J.; Hart, R.P.; Garrettson, L.K.; Stockman, S.; Hamer, R.M.; Schultz
     C.; Narasimhachari, N.: Post-traumatic stress disorder from pentaborane intoxica-
     tion: Neuropsychiatric evaluation and short term follow-up. J. Am. med. Ass. *254:*
     18, 2603–2608 (1985).

43   Robins, L.N.; Helzer, J.E.; Croughlin, J.; Ratcliffe, K.S.: National Institute of
     Mental Health Diagnostic Interview Schedule. Its history, characteristics and valid-
     ity. Archs gen. Psychiat. *38:* 381–389 (1981).

44   Lishman, W.A.; Ron, M.; Acker, W.: Computed tomography of the brain and
     psychometric assessment of alcoholic patients. A British study; in Sandler, Psycho-
     pharmacology of alcohol (Raven Press, New York 1980).

45   Weinberger, D.R.; DeLisi, L.E.; Perman, G.P.: CT scans in schizophreniform
     disorder and other acute psychiatric patients. Archs gen. Psychiat. *39:* 778–783
     (1982).

46   Levin, H.S.; Moyers, C.A.; Grossman, R.G.; Sarwar, M.: Ventricular enlargement
     after closed head injury. Archs Neurol. *33:* 623–629 (1981).

47   Hart, R.P.; Silverman, J.J.; Garrettson, L.K.; Hamer, R.M.: Neuropsychological
     function following mild exposure to pentaborane. Am. J. ind. Med. *6:* 37–44 (1984).

48   Pavlov, I.P.: In Anrep, Conditioned reflexes. An investigation of the physiologic
     activity of the cerebral cortex (1927) (Dover, New York 1960).

49   Dobbs, D.; Wilson, W.P.: Observations on persistence of war neurosis. Dis. nerv.
     Syst. *21:* 40–46 (1961).

50 Blanchard, E.B.; Kolb, L.C.; Pallmeyer, T.P.; Gerardi, R.J.: A psychophysiologic study of post-traumatic stress disorder in Viet Nam veterans. Psychiatry 54: 220–229 (1952).

51 Friedman, M.J.: Post-Vietnam syndrome. Recognition and management. Psychosomatics 22: 931–943 (1981).

52 Burstein, A.: Treatment of post-traumatic stress disorder with imipramine. Psychosomatics 25: 681–687 (1984).

53 Maier, S.F.; Seligman, M.E.T.: Learned helplessness. Theory and evidence. J. exp. Psychol. 105: 3–46 (1976).

54 Anisman, H.L.; Sklar, L.S.: Catecholamine depletion in mice upon reexposure to stress. Mediation of the escape deficits produced by inescapable shock. J. comp. Physiol. Psychol. 93: 610–625 (1979).

55 Anisman, H.L.; Ritch, M.; Sklar, L.S.: Noradrenergic and dopaminergic interactions in escape behavior. Analysis of uncontrollable stress effects. Psychopharm. Bull. 74: 263–268 (1981).

56 Kolk, B.: Post-traumatic stress disorder. Psychological and biological sequelae (American Psychiatric Press, Washington 1984).

57 Wise, M.G.: Post-traumatic stress disorder. The human reaction to catastrophe. Drug Ther. 3: 383–388 (1983).

58 Bowman, B.: The Vietnam veteran 10 years on. Aust. N.Z.J. Psychiat. 16: 107–127 (1982).

59 Lifton, R.J.: Home from the war: Viet Nam veterans. Neither victims nor executioners (Simon & Schuster, New York 1973).

60 Spiegel, D.: Vietnam grief work using hypnosis. Am. J. clin. Hypn. 24: 33–40 (1981).

61 Berger, D.M.: Survivors syndrome of problem of nosology and treatment. Am. J. Psychother. 31: 238–251 (1977).

62 Ewalt, J.R.; Crawford, D.: Post-traumatic stress syndrome. Curr. psychiat. Ther. 20: 145–153 (1981).

63 Rosenheim, E.; Elizur, A.: Group therapy for traumatic neurosis. Curr. psychiat. Ther. 16: 143–148 (1977).

64 Horowitz, M.: Stress response syndrome. Character style and dynamic psychotherapy. Archs gen. Psychiat. 31: 768–781 (1974).

65 Walker, J.I.; Cavenar, J.O.: Viet Nam veterans. Their problems continue. J. nerv. ment. Dis. 170: 174–180 (1982).

66 Burstein, A.: Treatment of post-traumatic stress disorder with imipramine. Psychosomatics 25: 681–687 (1984).

67 Lindy, J.D.; Grace, M.C.; Green, B.L.: Survivors. Outreach to a reluctant population. Am. J. Orthopsychiat. 51: 573–580 (1981).

68 Hogben, G.L.; Kornfield, R.B.: Treatment of traumatic neurosis with phenelzine. Archs gen. Psychiat. 38: 440–445 (1981).

69 Kolb, L.C.; Burris, B.C.; Griffiths, S.: Propranolol and quinidine in treatment of chronic post-traumatic stress disorders of war; in Van Der Kolk, Post-traumatic stress disorder: psychological and biological sequelae, chap. 6 (American Psychiatric Press, Washington 1984).

70 Pleading PTSD. Time May: 59 (1980).

71 Braverman, M.: Validity of psycho-traumatic reactions. J. forens. Sci. 22: 654–662 (1977).

72   Kelly, R.: The post-traumatic syndrome. An iatrogenic disease. Forens. Sci 6: 17–24 (1975).
73   Zilberg, N.J.; Weiss, D.S.; Horowitz, M.J.: Impact of even scale. A cross-validation study and some empirical evidence supporting a conceptual model of stress response syndrome. J. consult. clin. Psychol. 50: 407–414 (1982).

Joel J. Silverman, MD, Consultation-Liaison Psychiatry, Medical College of Virginia, Richmond, VA 23298 (USA)

Adv. psychosom. Med., vol. 16, pp. 141–152 (Karger, Basel 1986)

Chronic Pain and Trauma

James T. Kelley

Chronic Pain Unit, The University of Texas Medical School at Houston, Houston, Tex., USA

Historically, the relief of pain has been an important medical objective with as much emphasis as the diagnosis and treatment of disease. With the advent of major trauma centers and increasing rates of survival after major trauma, the relief of chronic pain has also increased in scope as a major medical problem. Protracted hospital and post-hospital courses, adjustment to loss of function, and acute, subacute and chronic pain all require adaptation; however, this adjustment process can be complicated by a number of physical and psychiatric factors. Anxiety states, depression, post-traumatic stress syndromes, and organic brain dysfunction all lead to less than adequate adjustment, prolonged recovery, disability and chronic pain syndromes. These factors can also lead to a chronic maladjustment that is out of proportion to the actual organic damage that the individual has suffered. The focus of this chapter will be on the psychiatric aspects of chronic maladjustment to pain following trauma. The complexity of the organic-psychogenic interaction in pain syndromes will be highlighted as opposed to the concept of dividing pain syndromes into strictly psychogenic or strictly organic. The role of early recognition, acknowledgement, and education regarding psychosocial adjustment to trauma in prevention or ameliorating chronic pain syndromes will be emphasized.

Chronic versus Acute Pain

The psychological and physical distinction between chronic and acute pain is at the root of many of the difficulties the medical profession has had in dealing with chronic pain syndromes. Physiologically, acute and chronic pain differ in the CNS pathways which are involved in pain transmission and different neurochemical systems may mediate these two processes [1]. In both chronic and acute pain, anxiety and depression magnify the subjective perception of pain, but in chronic pain syndromes this association is more intense. Perhaps the most important, but least recognized difference between acute and chronic pain are the necessary changes in role and expectations that evolve when dealing with chronic versus acute processes [2]. In acute illness or pain, the role of the patient and doctor are well defined. The patient is more passively dependent upon the physician to determine what is wrong and to prescribe treatment with which the patient is to comply. Dependence upon the physician is expected. In this model, the patient 'rightfully' expects the doctor to find the problem and solution to the immediate symptomatology. Society allows a person with acute illness to relinquish adult responsibility. If one is sick, one is excused from work, parenting and other adult responsibilities. When an illness becomes chronic, other role alterations occur. The goal is no longer one of alleviation of illness, but one of rehabilitation and coping with a chronic illness that cannot be cured. In a chronic process, this change in goals must be clearly understood by both physician and patient.

Rehabilitation requires the physician to assume a more passive role while the patient is more active in organizing, pursuing, and complying with various therapies to maintain health and function at an optimal level. Society's expectations also change as the individual must assume many adult responsibilities and is no longer totally free of adult obligations. A major focal point in all chronic maladjustment syndromes including the chronic pain syndrome is the lack of understanding by both patient and doctor of their roles [3]. Some patients only need to hear their problem defined as one with which they will have to learn to live as the medical profession has no cure. Once defined in this way, the patient will often adapt very quickly; however, continued evaluations and referrals to other physicians only serve to delay the adjustment process. Often the acceptance of the finality and reality of chronic physical dysfunction and pain is a difficult psychological process very much like bereavement. A variety of psychological responses to the news that ones ailment is chronic can be seen including denial, anger, depression, resistance, and excessive dependence. When dealt with honestly in the framework of the reality of the rehabilitation effort, the patient can do relatively well in working through these processes.

The patient's difficulties in accepting the reality of a chronic process are paralleled by the physician. At times, doctors may have difficulty in accepting the fact that their skills have very little to offer a particular patient. Underlying this difficulty are issues of competence, self-esteem, and ominipotence which are challenged when cures are not forthcoming. More often, the physician's difficulties in accepting the reality of a chronic disease syndrome are secondary to an over-identification with the patient's plight. Thus, the doctor colludes with the patient to avoid the reality of the chronic situation to save them both from the psychological pain. The simplicity of this concept greatly belies its importance.

A frank discussion of the roles and expectations of the patient and physician is the starting point of the patient's learning to deal with chronic pain or dysfunction. The patient often has to be repeatedly told about these roles and expectations for what seems to be understood one day, will be totally repressed the next. Family members also need to understand the goals and expectations of this effort. It is not uncommon to have a chronic pain syndrome prolonged, not because a patient cannot accept the chronicity of his problem, but because an important family member cannot give up the myth that a cure is imminent.

The Placebo Effect

The earliest known and used successful medical treatment must surely have been the placebo effect. This effect is seen when a patient has a decrease in symptomatology after treatment, be it a pill or some procedure, when given by an authoritative figure. If the patient has a strong positive expectation, indeed the treatment will alleviate the symptoms. As the understanding of complex organic-psychogenic etiologies of many clinical syndromes became apparent to physicians, the placebo effect mistakenly became equated with psychogenic etiology. This does not stand up to scientific study. Anxiety has been shown to consistently decrease pain threshold whether or not neurotic tendencies are present [4]. Additional studies also suggest a role of endorphins in this response [5]. Evidence for placebo effect does not then mean that an individual's pain is psychogenic.

Efforts to tease apart organic and psychogenic issues often exceed their clinical utility. Most pain patient have a complex intermingling of organic and psychological features. An expectation by the physician that psychological factors are important in every patient coping with pain in the acute or chronic phase is extremely valuable.

Pain as Communication

As stated above, acute physical pain is one of the few situations in which society will allow a person to honorably relinquish his adult responsibilities. Likewise, societies and families are much more tolerant to a person's distress, if it is physical pain. Anxiety, depression, and psychological pain are less acceptable symptoms to both society and the individual. This tendency for physical pain to be a successful method of communicating distress and alleviating one's responsibility as opposed to the emotional symptoms that accompany pain is in part culturally determined [see article by *Gaines*, this vol.]. Clearly, people with chronic pain are apt to use this acceptable communication of distress to complain when quite possibly the most distressing issues relate to loss of self-esteem and anxiety about financial problems. Likewise, a great temptation exists for the individual to use his physical pain as an excuse to avoid situations which increase his anxiety. While this is in part related to social approval and psychological conservation, a physiologic exacerbation of pain can evolve as the individual approaches the situation which increases emotional tension and increases his perception of pain. Patient education and physician recognition of this phenomenon are very important. More complex associations between pain complaints and psychological distress exist. Pain may be the only way an individual can express his distress about unresolved grief over the death of a loved one [see article by *Brown,* this vol.]. Pain can also be a way of expressing anger over past relationships.

The evolution of chronic pain generally involves multiples of such factors. Often in any one given individual, an equilibrium has developed between the stresses of daily life and the patient's mechanisms of defense. When the person is involved with acute illness or trauma, this stress overtaxes the coping systems that have developed and simultaneously offers a psychologically acceptable way of communicating a number of distresses and reduces the responsibility that the individual must incur. As this evolves, reduction of pain not only becomes a function of organic tissue factors, but also a function of the patient's present and past conflicts. Education regarding the emotional aspects of pain is extremely important. In most pain patients, the emphasis should be placed on the fact that the pain is not imaginary or 'in their head', but that the pain is real and is directly influenced by emotional state.

Specific Psychiatric Symptoms Associated with Chronic Pain

Post-Traumatic Stress Syndrome

As discussed in the paper by *Silverman* [this vol.], one of the major psychiatric complications of trauma can be post-traumatic stress syndrome. This by definition is a highly anxious state and therefore increases the patient's perception of pain. More importantly, however, is how the person interprets these symptoms. Often, anxiety, panic, and phobic symptomatology are perceived as signs of weakness and are often unable to be acknowledged as significant impediments to recovery. Many patients find it easier to complain of the somatic symptom of pain and to use these symptoms to avoid the phobic situation which often relates to work. This process has been observed in heavy machine accidents, scaffold workers, and in a variety of drivers that were involved in work-related accidents. These people can be quickly maligned by the professionals' feeling that all they really want is to avoid work and receive disability. Exacerbation of pain symptomatology or combinations of anxiety mixed with pain following trauma which permits the avoidance of the anxiety-provoking situation, should suggest the possibility of PTSD. Once diagnosed, education is very important. *Silverman's* paper [this vol.] outlines many direct intervention strategies which are useful.

Depression

The losses that occur with trauma lead directly to dysphoria and depression [see article by *Brown,* this vol.]. Chronic pain as an irritative stimuli produces difficulties with sleeping and chronic fatigue. This irritability also leads to isolation and withdrawal. Sexual dysfunction and disability can lead to difficulties with self-esteem. Depression is associated with increased subjective awareness of pain [4]. Attempts to minimize the impact of this decreased self-esteem makes the patient vulnerable to maximizing physical symptoms to increase self-worth and communicate distress.

Depression should be suspected in all cases of chronic post-traumatic pain. The classic neurovegetative symptoms of depression should be evaluated: loss of appetite, sleep disturbance (especially early morning awakening), diurnal variation of mood, loss of energy and interest, feelings of helplessness or hopelessness, crying spells, suicidal ideation. In pain patients, these symptoms are often explained away as secondary to pain. Education about loss and depression are very important components in treatment as well as psychotherapy and pharmacotherapy. A number of antidepressants (amitriptyline, doxepin and trazodone) have been used in the treatment of chronic pain and depression [4, 6]. The neuropharmacology of these agents suggests both an analgesic and antidepressant effect.

Substance Abuse

Drug and alcohol abuse are major causes of trauma and can also become a major problem afterward [see article by *Reilly* et al., this vol.]. If a substance dependence problem was involved in the trauma, it will certainly be a difficult problem that can lead to major difficulties in the post traumatic adjustment period. If persistent pain is a problem post trauma, a number of patients will start to abuse narcotics and/or alcohol for pain control. On a chronic basis, the use of narcotics and alcohol leads to tolerance and depression as well as to problems with cognitive functioning, sleep disturbance, and fatigue which can lead to lower self-esteem and decreased pain threshold. Substance dependence can quickly become the most disabling condition and provoke an increase in pain behavior. A subclinical organic brain syndrome can also accompany significant drug or alcohol abuse and predispose the individual to the use of more primitive defense mechanisms such as denial and projection. These occurrences reinforce the use of somatization and increase the unwillingness to consider drugs and alcohol as primary difficulties.

In general, the first order of business is the establishment and maintenance of a substance-free state. Then depression can be properly evaluated over time. The education of the chronic pain patient to the medical facts about chronic substance dependence is very important. The fact that tolerance and withdrawal are physiological givens with extended narcotic use must be repeatedly stressed. The physician must be persistent in getting this point across to both patient and family.

Chronic Pain Syndrome

The chronic pain syndrome is defined as a pain state that persists daily over 6 months in which conventional surgical and medical treatment are unsuccessful. The patient finds the symptomatology disabling and the severity of symptoms seems out of proportion to the actual tissue damage observed. In this section we will focus on the early stages of chronic pain, that is 6 months to 2 years. Once a patient has had a pain problem over 6 months, it is safe to assume that a protracted problem is developing. At this point addressing the chronic pain issue is critical. Even in the well-prepared patient, the reality of chronicity can precipitate depression or anxiety. These responses must be dealt with through education, psychotherapy and even psychotropics, if neurovegetative signs of depression become evident. Once a pain state becomes chronic, there is going to be an ebb and flow of physical and psychological symptomatology. Often, patients will seem to be adjusting quite well for a period of months or years, but a major stress in their life (like divorce or loss of a job) can provoke a reemergence of symptoms. Continuing education and support is necessary for most chronic pain patients. Vocational questions must be addressed early in the treatment process. If it is likely the patient will have to be retained, education and counselling about this as early as possible can be quite helpful. Despite the fact that chronic pain conditions are not always preventable, early comprehensive treatment post-trauma can significantly aid in making the chronic pain patient as functional as possible.

Stages of Pain

Hendler [7] and others have divided the psychological response to pain into four stages. These stages are similar to those that *Kubler-Ross* [8] has outlined as the normal response to death and dying. The four stages of pain as outlined by *Hendler* can be adapted to the recovering trauma patient. This will encompass much of what has already been stated, but will incorporate educational, emotional, and psychological variables of a pain syndrome into a fairly specific guide for the clinician in developing a treatment approach to the trauma patient.

Acute Pain

Acute pain may be described as that which the trauma patient encounters in the first 2 months post-trauma. This stage, especially the first 2–4 weeks, has caused a fair amount of controversy in clinical treatment of pain. A number of authors have strongly stated that the medical profession's fear of addiction and general feeling that the 'good patient' suffers pain without complaint has led the physician to grossly undermedicate people in acute pain with much disruption of patient/doctor relationship [9]. This school of thought has a number of very salient points especially when one looks at acute pain, postoperative pain, and pain from progressive malignant disease. The key issue here is the use of narcotic analgesics. The intelligent use of narcotics and education about their effects on the patient in the acute pain stage is a very important step in limiting the development of a chronic pain syndrome. The attitude of giving as little narcotics as possible by the medical system in the acute pain stage may actually lead to more problems with narcotic abuse and dependence in the majority of patients. As outlined by *Hackett* [9], using less than adequate narcotic dosages and lengthy time intervals between dosages will often increase the patient's anxiety and heighten pain. The conflict and hostility that can be generated by not giving narcotics for pain can destroy trust and the patient's willingness to believe any of what the physician will tell him about pain management. When an argument regarding the amount of narcotic erupts between patient and staff, the patient's feelings of loss of control and decrease in self-esteem heighten. The physician who liberally uses narcotics in the acute pain period with proper education as to their short-term role and the problems that these drugs can have, may find that his patient will see him as a true ally in the battle against pain. Later, when the physician states that there is a time when the patient should not take narcotics, but should find other ways to deal with pain, as well as to accept that dealing with pain will have to be a day-in, day-out experience, he will be believed much more readily.

Patients who have been undermedicated in acute pain may harbor resentment and hostility toward the physician in the sense that the physician never really understood or was interested in helping them deal with their pain. Education about narcotics, their short-term and long-term effects and about the emotional aspects of recovering from severe trauma are the key to the use of narcotics in the acute phase post-trauma. Much emphasis should be placed on the patient (except in organic brain syndromes) being primarily responsible for monitoring his pain during this period. *Hackett's* guidelines of ordering pain medication every three or four hours except if the patient refuses allows for a p.r.n. management of pain, but without putting the nursing staff in the judgemental role of real versus nonreal pain. As the patient increases his autonomy and also his self-esteem, anxiety decreases and a strengthened therapeutic alliance emerges. By educating the patient as to the time and indication parameters of narcotic use, this alliance is further promoted. He should be educated as to the development of tolerance and withdrawal and that excessive use of narcotics will destabilize sleep patterns, leading to fatigue and depression which increase pain perception.

Another important area in the acute stage of the post-trauma patient is the discussion about the extent of an individual's injury and his potential for recovery. Somewhat akin to patients with terminal illness, trauma patients usually want to know what is going to happen to their bodies. Some will not be able to bear the truth about the extent of their injuries early in the course of recovery, but most want to hear the reality of their condition. The physician should answer these questions honestly and the unknown should be handled directly.

The patient should be informed that depression, anger and resentment typically emerge post-trauma, but that they do not signal mental illness. Techniques which facilitate the patient's verbalizations regarding his emotional state will prevent pain symptoms and medication from becoming a means of communicating and/or mediating anxiety and depression. Even when the patient denies these feeling states, which is often the case, it is important to educate the patient about them. This prepares the patient and opens the door for his physician if overt difficulties occur.

On occasion, a patient will tenaciously hold on to a false belief about recovery. For example, a patient might have strong beliefs that he might eventually have the use of a limb when basically the prognosis is guarded. This patient will hold onto this belief despite the physician humanely telling him that chances are poor for any extended recovery of function. Often patients need to hold on to this belief in order to avoid intense depression or anxiety. Confrontation of this type of denial is not requisite unless it becomes a stumbling block in terms of motivation in a rehabilitation program. If the use of denial reduces anxiety and allows appropriate function, no intervention is indicated. If it becomes, 'well, I'm going to wait until my limb is better or the pain is less, to work with the physical therapy, etc.', then more active confrontation is needed.

A summary or outline of pain management for acute stage would be as follows: (1) Give as much autonomy as possible. (2) Educate about the short-term use of narcotics and how pain management will change if the pain continues past 1 or 2 months. (3) After 1 month, only oral medications should be used with the daily use of narcotics never extending beyond 6 months. (4) Educate about grief and emotional aspects of pain and how these emotions are normal although they may intensify pain. (5) Use psychotropic treatment if severe anxiety and depression develops. (6) Vigorously treat post-traumatic stress syndrome if it develops.

Sub-Acute Pain

The sub-acute pain stage as defined by Hendler exists from 2 to 6 months post-trauma. *Hendler* [7] feels that the normal response of patients during this period is to continue to have a certain amount of denial, but that one also sees the development of anxiety or depression. These may be manifested as irritability with family, problems with sleep, increased perception of pain and possibly renewed use or increased use of narcotic analgesics, alcohol or tranquilizers. This is a crucial time for the patient. During this period the groundwork *will be laid for the type of adjustment* and coping mechanisms that will be used throughout recovery. An objective and frank approach about the long-term outcome for the patient is important. The risks and benefits of any medical or surgical intervention should be discussed truthfully with the patient. Dynamic differences between chronic and acute pain should be discussed. Narcotics, alcohol, and illicit drug use have to be curtailed during this period and dealt with openly.

In this stage ancillary measures for pain management are often necessary. The use of tricyclic antidepressants alone or in combination with neuroleptics can be helpful for pain management, even in the absence of extreme anxiety or depression. The use of anticonvulsants for central pain states alone or in combination with neuroleptics or tricyclics can be helpful for pain management, even in the absence of extreme anxiety or depression. Physical therapy, massage, and t.e.n.s. units can be useful during this time. Other techniques such as biofeedback and relaxation training can be used as adjunctive aids to the individual who is having trouble managing pain. At this point depression and anxiety are more apparent in family members of the patient. Their education regarding prognosis, the medical system, and the patient's needs relative to pain and disability is extremely important. Education of the family concerning problems of addictive drugs is also essential.

We have experienced mixed results in treating patients during this stage of recovery on a chronic pain unit. At times the medical unknowns and ongoing procedures preclude the patient's developing the emotional and cognitive states necessary to utilize ancillary modalities for pain management. Success has been better in situations where patients are having a fair degree of anxiety and depression and when medical/surgical procedures are relatively limited. Guidelines for treatment of pain in the sub-acute period post-trauma are as follows:

(1) Look closely for signs of depression and anxiety that are not being verbalized.

(2) Opiate use should be on the decline (even in hospitalized patients): nondaily use of narcotics is the goal.

(3) Continuing education about the normality of a variety of emotions during this stage of recovery, educating the patient's family about the hazards of long-term addictive drug use, and education about the patient/family responsibilities dealing with a more chronic process is needed.

(4) Ancillary measures for pain management are introduced including anticonvulsants, neuroleptics, antidepressants, biofeedback, relaxation techniques and physical therapy.

References

1   Hendler, N.: The anatomy and psychopharmacology of pain. J. clin. Psychiat. *43:* 14–20 (1982).

2   DeVaul, R.A.; Zisook, S.; Stuart, H.U.: Patients with psychogenic pain. J. fam. Pract. *4:* 53–55 (1977).

3   DeVaul, R.A.; Zisook, S.: Chronic pain! The psychiatrists role. Psychosomatics *19:* 417–421 (1978).

4   Halpern, C.: Substitution-detoxification and its role in the management of chronic benign pain. J. clin. Psychiat. *43:* 10–15.

5   Levine, J.D.; Gordon, N.C.; Fields, H.L.: The mechanism of placebo analgesia. Lancet *1978:* 654–667.

6   Hameroff, S.R.; Cork, R.C.; Scherer, K.; Crago, B.R.; Neuman, C.; Womble, J.R.; Davis, T.P.: Doxepine effects on chronic pain, depression and plasma opioids. J. clin. Psychiat. *48:* 22–27 (1982).

7   Hendler, N.: The four stages of pain; in Hendler, Diagnosis and treatment of chronic pain, pp. 1–19 (Wright, Massachusetts).

8   Kubler-Ross, E.: On death and dying (McMillan, New York 1979).

9   Hackett, T.P.: We've got to do more for patients in pain. Med. Econ. *Jan:* 113–122 (1976).

James T. Kelley, MD, Chronic Pain Unit, The University of Texas Medical School at Houston, Houston, TX 77004 (USA)

Adv. psychosom. Med., vol. 16, pp. 153–172 (Karger, Basel 1986)

Descriptive Epidemiologic Studies of Head Injury in the United States: 1974–1984[1]

Ralph F. Frankowski

University of Texas, School of Public Health, Houston, Tex., USA

The prerequisite in studying a disease is its definition. In the broadest sense, head injury refers to acute physical damage of the face, scalp, skull, dura, or brain caused by external mechanical (kinetic) energy. Head injuries may be classified according to the structure involved. The scalp alone may be injured, or the skull may be fractured. Within the skull, either the dura or the brain itself, or both may be damaged. Depending on the type and degree of the external force, any of these injuries may be present alone or in any combination.

Most head injuries, such as contusions, lacerations, or simple fractures are inconsequential to the individual. The individual recovers from such head injuries uneventfully, without significant sequelae. However, other head injuries which alone or in combination affect or threaten the organic integrity of the brain may result in serious morbidity. Injury to the brain may result in death or cause significant, and possibly irreversible neurological, neuropsychological, or functional impairments. Brain damage as a consequence of head injuries is the event of medical and epidemiologic interest [1].

Prior to 1980, the only published information available about the occurrence of head injury for the population of the United States was that gathered by the National Center for Health Statistics in its Health Interview Survey [2]. The National Health Interview Survey (NHIS) is a continuous nationwide sample survey in which data are collected through personal household interviews. The universe for NHIS is the civilian noninstitutionalized population of the United States. The usual

[1] This research was supported in part by NIH-NINCDS contract NO1-NS-9-2314B.

NHIS sample is about 111,000 persons in 41,000 households a year. An injured person is defined by NHIS as anyone having suffered an injury in an accident or in intentional violence, and who is medically attended or whose activity is limited, or both, for at least one full day.

Information from the National Health Interview Survey provided the first national estimates of the frequency of head injury in the United States. *Caveness* [3] estimated that for the time period 1970 to 1976, head injuries accounted for 12% of 65 million injuries reported by NHIS. About 4% of the population of the United States annually reported some type of head injury. Head injuries were classified as either mild or major [3]. Mild injuries included lacerations of the head, and contusions of the scalp, face, and neck. Major head injuries included concussions, skull fractures, and intracranial injuries. The majority, about 3 of every 4 head injuries reported, were mild injuries. However, the remainder were classified as major injuries with the potential for brain injury. For the period 1970 to 1976 more than one million major head injuries per year were reported for the population of the United States [3].

The NHIS head injury data are subject to a number of limitations. The data on injuries are self-reported and thus lack clinical confirmation. The data include self-treated injuries as well as medically-treated injuries; new injuries are not distinguished from previous injuries, and the extent of recall bias is unknown. Yet, despite the limitations of the NHIS data, the potential magnitude of the health problem of head injuries is substantial. Head injuries appear to be commonplace and not infrequently severe.

The NHIS data on head injuries prompted a series of independent investigations to obtain more refined estimates on the occurrence of head injury in the United States. The surveys attempted to answer, for defined populations, who sustained head injuries, the type and severity of the head injuries, as well as when and where injuries occur, and why. These inquiries form the basis of the descriptive epidemiology of head injury, the topic of this chapter.

Frequency and Rates of Head Injury

Incidence and prevalence are two common measures of the frequency of head injury for a defined population. Prevalence is the proportion of a defined population affected by head injury at a specified point in time. The numerator of the proportion is all persons in a population affected by head injury at that instant, regardless of whether the head injury was recent or in the distant past. Incidence refers to new cases of head injury, both fatal and nonfatal, occurring among previously unaffected individuals of a defined population. Rates, in contrast, require the dimension of time. The annual incidence rate for a particular population and calendar year is the number of new cases of head injury ascertained during the year, divided by an approximation of the total amount of risk-time of the population, usually the size of the midyear population. The denominator estimates the number in the population at risk of a head injury and previously unaffected. Head injury incidence rates are commonly expressed as head injuries per 100,000 population per year.

The first specialized survey of the frequency and rates of head injury for the United States population was the National Head and Spinal Cord Injury Survey [4] conducted under the auspices of the National Institute of Neurological and Communicative Disorders and Stroke. The head injury survey objectives were to estimate the occurrence of new cases, the frequency of existing cases, their demographic correlates, the causes of head injury, and the economic costs of head injury for the population of the contiguous United States for the year 1974. Head injury was defined as physical injury to the brain caused by an external (mechanical) force, including birth trauma. The survey population for head injury consisted of persons who had received inpatient hospital care for the treatment of a head injury during the time period 1970 through 1974. Head injury deaths that did not receive inpatient hospital care were excluded from the survey.

In the National Head and Spinal Cord Injury Survey the occurrence of head injury was measured by enumeration of hospital admission and discharge records. The operational definition of a case of head injury was based on a pre-defined set of standard hospital diagnostic codes that referred to conditions indicative of direct injury to the brain. The diagnostic codes were selected from the standard medical nomenclature used by hospitals for describing clinical and pathological observations as prescribed in the Eighth Revision, International Classification of Diseases, Adapted for Use in the United States (HICDA) [5]. The set of primary head injury codes included all HICDA codes for intracranial injuries and select traumatic brain injury codes associated with mental disorders. This primary set of 13 HICDA codes was supplemented by a set of 13 additional HICDA diagnostic codes that were thought to be frequently associated with brain injury but were not in themselves indicative of brain injury, e.g. skull fractures. Such cases were included only if the medical records of the case contained evidence of neurologic signs or symptoms of brain injury [4].

The National Head and Spinal Cord Injury Survey was a multistage national probability survey with three section stages. The first stage of random selection was 58 geographic areas from 1,675 areas covering the United States. The second stage selected a total of 305 hospitals from within the 58 geographic areas, and the third stage consisted of a sample of patient records from each of the hospitals selected in the second stage. More than 200,000 eligible discharges were listed and approximately 10,000 selected for case ascertainment. The participation rate of hospitals was 81%, and 93% of the hospital records were found suitable for review and analysis. Health cost interviews were also completed for 609 of 913 patients who had sustained either a head or spinal cord injury in 1974.

The major findings of the National Head and Spinal Cord Injury Survey were surprising. For the United States population in 1974, the rate of hospitalization for incident head injuries was estimated at 200 per 100,000 population; 422,000 new hospitalized cases of head injury occurred in 1974. The rates of occurrence of head injury did not vary significantly among geographic regions. Over the time period 1970 through 1974, the average number of new cases of head injury hospitalized each year in the United States was about 400,000, a figure estimated with a relative standard error of 7.2% [6]. The frequency of existing cases of head injury in the United States population for 1974, as judged by the number of rehospitalizations for head injuries, was twice the rate of occurrence for new injuries. A total of 926,000 cases of head injuries, first occurring in the years 1970 through 1974 still required hospital treatment and readmission in 1974. For the total population in 1974, direct-care plus indirect costs associated with head injury were $2.4 billion [6].

The range of severity of injuries ascertained in the National Survey was unknown. However, the survey estimated, within the limitation of the diagnostic codes, the frequency of the major types of injuries found. About 75% of the new injuries were concussions, 6% were cerebral lacerations or contusions, and 2% were hematomas. The percentage of patients who died during the first hospital stay after head injury in 1974 was 3.0%, with a relative standard error of 20.3% [6].

The National Health Interview Survey and the National Head and Spinal Cord Injury Survey produced an interesting contrast about the occurrence of head injury in the United States. Self-reported major head injuries were three times more frequent than observed hospital admissions for similar major head injuries. Although the differences in definitions and case ascertainment between the two national surveys likely explain much of this discrepancy, the broad implications of the calculus of head injury remained; somewhat more than one million persons in the United States in 1974 required inpatient hospital care for the treatment of new or old acute head injuries.

The national information indicated clearly that head injury was a major cause of morbidity in the United States yet descriptive epide-miologic studies of the incidence of head injury in specific commu-nities or populations lagged. The logistics of population-based ascer-tainment of head injuries are exacting, expensive, and time-consuming. Difficulties in identifying and uniquely classifying cases are sub-stantial, and the lack of standardized definitions, clinical criteria, and mutually-exclusive hospital diagnostic categories deterred many investigators. As a result most of the published data during the decade 1970–1980 on the frequency head injury emanated from reports of case series of hospital admissions without reference to a population base [7]. A notable exception occurred with the publication of a report on the incidence, causes, and secular trends of head trauma for the population of Olmsted County, Minn. for the period 1935 through 1974 [8].

The setting for this remarkable investigation was the unique pop-ulation-based medical records linkage system of the Rochester Project at the Mayo Clinic, a medical surveillance system designed to study the population occurrence of a number of diagnosed diseases, particularly neurological disorders. *Annegers* et al. [8] took advantage of this data resource to study and clarify many of the issues about the population occurrence of head injury. The Mayo Research Group departed from case-finding based on HICDA diagnostic codes, as used in the National Head and Spinal Cord Injury Survey, and based their definition of head trauma instead on clinical criteria of brain injury. Head trauma was defined as head injury with evidence of presumed brain involvement.

The clinical criteria required evidence of concussion with loss of consciousness (LOC), posttraumatic amnesia (PTA), or neurological signs of brain injury. Skull fractures, however, were included, even without altered consciousness [8]. Incident cases of head injury were derived from hospital admissions, emergency room visits, out-patient examinations, and home visits. All county death certificates and autopsy protocols were also reviewed. Approximately 40,000 records from the time period 1935 through 1974 were reviewed. Case ascertainment of medically-treated cases of head trauma should have been virtually complete for the Olmsted County population. Employing the general clinical criteria of LOC, PTA, confirmed brain injury, or skull fracture to define cases of head injury, the 1965–1974 age-adjusted mean annual incidence rate per 100,000 population for Olmsted County was estimated at 270 among males and 116 among females. Fatal head injuries accounted for 13% of the total male incidence rate and 9% of the total female incidence rate [8].

The Olmsted County study was followed in rapid succession by reports of the incidence of head injury in the populations of Bronx County, New York; San Diego County, Calif.; North Central Virginia, and select communities of the Chicago area. The Bronx County study [9] of 1980 and the Chicago area study [10] of 1979–1980 employed definitions and case ascertainment procedures similar to those used in the Olmsted County Study. Incidence for the Bronx County population for the year 1980 was reported at 249 head injuries per 100,000 population. Fatal head injuries accounted for 11% of the total Bronx incidence rate. The incidence rates for the Chicago area communities of Evanston, Ill., and a small inner-city Chicago population were estimated at 215 among Evanston whites, 454 for the inner city community blacks, and 575 for Evanston blacks. Fatal head injuries accounted for about 5% of the total head injury incidence in the Chicago area surveys but the incidence rates are unstable due to small numbers of cases.

Patients with documented head injuries who were admitted to a regional medical center serving a 12 county rural area of North Central Virginia produced for the year 1978 [11]. Nearly all cases had one or more of the conditions of LOC, PTA, or skull fracture. However, the case series excluded non-hospital deaths and cases not referred to the regional medical center thus this incidence estimate is not strictly population-based.

Two epidemiologic surveys have described the frequency of head injury for the population of San Diego County, Calif., for the years 1978 and 1981. The 1978 survey [12] was a population study of all deaths due to head injury and of all patients admitted to San Diego hospitals with a diagnosis of head injury, excluding gunshot wounds. Diagnoses were based on HICDA codes identifying cases of skull fractures or intracranial injuries as recorded in a common data base of San Diego hospital admissions and discharges. For the year 1978 the total incidence of head injury, including possibly cases with non-neurologic head injuries and injuries to non-residents, was 295/100,000 population. Fatal head injuries excluding gunshot wounds accounted for 8% of the total incidence rate.

The 1981 San Diego County study [13] provided incidence rates of acute brain injury by restricting cases to individuals whose medical records had physician-diagnosed and confirmed evidence of brain injury. The study excluded persons with skull or facial bone fracture or soft tissue damage not accompanied by evidence of brain injury. Cases of presumed brain involvement were thereby excluded. The casefinding protocol was based on a list of 12 HICDA admission codes that were likely to capture most cases of acute brain injury. Case ascertainment was accomplished by review of emergency room and hospital records, coroners' cases, death certificates, nursing home records, and local emergency medical transport records. The estimated 1981 annual incidence rate of physician-confirmed acute brain injury for San Diego County was 180/100,000 population. Fatal head injuries from all causes accounted for 12% of the total incidence of acute brain injury [13].

Research on the population-based frequency of head injury has set as its goal the enumeration of the specific extent of fatal and nonfatal brain injury in defined communities. However, case-finding and case-ascertainment procedures of studies vary considerably, as well as attention to the full diagnostic spectrum of actual or presumed brain injury. As a result the exact measurement of risk of brain injury is confounded with study methodologies and population characteristics. Any generalizations are therefore tenuous. From the information to date, if brain injury is taken as evident intracranial injury, skull fracture, or head injury accompanied with loss of consciousness or posttraumatic amnesia then incidence rates for large heterogeneous US population groups range from somewhat less than 0.2–0.3% per year. Approximately 10% of the incident brain injuries are fatal.

Demographic Correlates and Causes of Head Injury

Two general demographic observations dominate all population reports on the incidence of head injury. Males are at least twice as likely as females to sustain a head injury (table I). Head injury incidence is also markedly elevated among young adults and among the elderly.

Age and gender are pervasive demographic factors associated with the incidence of head injury. Male age-specific incidence is greater than female incidence throughout the entire age span. The most pronounced separation of male and female incidence occurs at ages 15–24 where the ratio of male to female incidence approaches 3.0. The least difference occurs at ages 0–4 where male incidence is only slightly in excess of female incidence [8–13].

Although methodological differences among studies preclude exact numerical comparisons of age-specific incidence rates, the patterns of incidence among studies are quite similar and illustrate the influence of age and gender on the occurrence of head injury. In the early years of life male incidence increases nearly uniformly to its absolute maximum at about age 20. Thereafter, male incidence declines to its absolute minimum at about age 55. At age 70 male incidence increases rapidly.

Table I Incidence of head injury as reported in selected studies by sex per 100,000 population per year

Population and year	Source	Sex	Incidence	Male/female ratio
United States (1974)	[6][1]	male	272	2.1
		female	132	
Olmsted County (1965–1974)	[8][2]	male	270	2.3
		female	116	
Bronx County (1980)	[9][2]	male	391	2.8
		female	142	
San Diego County (1981)	[13][3]	male	247	2.2
		female	111	

[1] Excludes nonhospital deaths.
[2] Includes all skull fractures, LOC or PTA cases.
[3] Confirmed acute brain injury only.

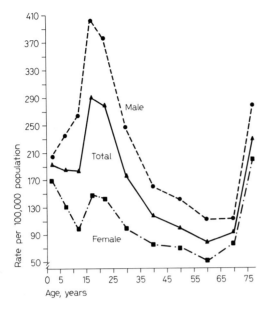

Fig. 1. Age- and sex-specific incidence rates of acute brain injury per 100,000 population, San Diego County, Calif., 1981 [from *Kraus* et al., 13; reproduced with permission of the authors and publishers].

In contrast, female incidence declines throughout the first decade of life but pivots at age 10 to peak at age 20. Female incidence then declines to age 60 or so and then rapidly increases again. Figure 1 illustrates the sex-age incidence for acute brain injury. The incidence patterns suggest that male and female incidence differs both in degree and kind. *Kraus* et al. [13] noted that nearly 70% of all acute brain injury cases were male.

Age incidence curves among populations are determined by two major factors: (1) the extent of exposure of the population to the causes of head injury, and (2) the congruence of ascertainment methods used to enumerate head injuries. Given the magnitude and extent of most populations to the injury hazards of transportation it comes as no surprise that means of transportation are the leading, proximate causes of head injury, regardless of case ascertainment methods. Recalling that the National Head and Spinal Cord Injury Survey excluded nonhospital deaths, table II shows that for the national population motor

Table II. Percent distribution of proximate causes of head injury as reported in selected studies

Population and year	Source	Transportation %	Falls %	Assault %	Recreation %	All other %	n
United States (1974)	[6]	49	28	NR	NR	23	1,210
Olmsted County (1935–1974)	[8]	46	29	7	9	9	3,587
Bronx County (1980)	[9]	27	32	34	NR	7	1,209
Evanston, Ill. (1980)	[10]						
Black		32	21	26	11	10	62
White		39	31	10	14	6	103
Inner-city Chicago (1980)	[10]						
Black		31	20	40	3	6	617
San Diego County (1981) (acute brain injury)	[13]	48	21	18	10	4	3,358

NR = Not reported.

vehicle crashes are responsible for at least ½ of all head injuries. This fraction is repeated in the causes of head injury for the affluent and geographically dispersed populations of Olmsted County and San Diego County.

Detailed data on transportation-related causes comes from the 1981 San Diego survey. Of 1,611 acute brain injuries owed to transportation, nearly ⅔ were sustained by occupants of motor vehicles. Motorcycle crashes accounted for nearly 20% of all transportation-related brain injuries. Motor vehicle-pedestrian accidents caused 12% of the head injuries and motor vehicle-bicyclist accidents 6% [13].

Falls explain approximately 20% to 30% of head injury incidence across all populations (see table II). Incidence from falls of all types among males exceeds female incidence at all ages [13]. The typical age-incidence curve due to falls follows a U shape where incidence is highest below age 5 and among those aged 65 and older. Falls are the major cause of head injury in the very young and the very old. *Whitman* et al. [10] observed an excess risk of total head injury in the first year of life compared to subsequent incidence to age 5. A finding that was not sought in other studies.

Assault explains 7% to 40% of all incident head injury (see table II). The risk of assault, given the limited data available, appears to be population dependent. The compressed and poor urban areas of Bronx and innercity Chicago show assault, transportation and falls as nearly equal causes of head injury. In the Bronx County, assault accounted for ⅓ of all cases of head injury. It was the most frequent cause of head injury among males of all races, affecting males four times as often as females [9]. Similar findings characterize the Chicago area studies [10].

Recreation-related injuries were reported as causes of 3–14% of head injuries among the populations. There is little uniformity in the classification of such injuries so that specific forms of sports and recreational activities cannot be uniquely identified. Since exposure to sports and recreation would be expected to vary substantially among populations their role in the incidence of head injury must be assessed by special studies of risk groups. Contact sports such as boxing, football, soccer, and rugby are not infrequently the cause of head injury with presumed brain involvement [1]. *Kraus* et al. [13] point out that organized sports, pedal cycles, roller skates, and skate boards accounted for 10% of all acute brain injuries in San Diego County. The insidious aspect of sports that may cause repeated concussions to participants is that the effects of repeated concussions are cumulative [1, 14].

Severity of Head Injury

Mortality data have certain important advantages in describing the frequency of a disease. In the United States deaths are completely enumerated, and each death is ascribed to an underlying cause of death by rules set forth in the International Classification of Disease. The convention for assigning causes of death to injuries is to classify such deaths by the circumstances of the accident or violence that produced the fatal injury. Although death certificates also contain standard information on the pathologies or nature of injuries, this information is not routinely reported at the national level.

In 1984 the National Center for Health Statistics released the first national tabulations on the nature of injuries reported on death certificates [15]. The report concerned deaths recorded for the year 1978. Injuries were reported for 211,000 of nearly 2 million deaths for 1978.

The category, intracranial injury (N850–N854), was reported for 50,000 deaths. (This category excludes skull fracture.) Conservatively, about 1 of every 4 deaths for the year 1978 involved an intracranial injury. Death certificate mention of intracranial injury was three times more frequent among males than females. About one-fourth of all intracranial injury deaths occurred to persons aged 15–24 [15].

The risk of death due to head injury has been estimated in most of the population studies of the incidence of head injury. Although the definition of a death due to head injury varies somewhat among studies age-adjusted death rates for large US communities are in the narrow range of 22–32 head injury deaths per 100,000 population [8, 9, 12, 13].

The general demographic features of head injury mortality can be illustrated by a 1980 three-county study of all deaths due to head injury [16]. Head injury deaths were ascertained for 1980 from among all fatal injuries that occurred to residents of Bronx County, New York; Harris County (Houston), Tex.; and San Diego County, Calif. Individuals whose fatal injuries included skull fracture, intracranial injury, and brain penetrating injury were identified. Properly speaking, all deaths involving an actual or probable brain injury were included in the survey.

When averaged across the counties, head injuries were present in one-third of all deaths from accidents and violence. The county age-adjusted death rates per 100,000 population ranged from 27 (Bronx County), 28 (San Diego County) to 31 (Harris County). Males had a risk of head injury mortality four times that of females (table III).

The age-adjusted head injury death rates for the three counties are quite similar, but the causes of the fatal injuries varied considerably among the counties (table III). Approximately, 40% of the head injury deaths in Bronx and Harris Counties were the result of gunshot wounds. The contribution of self-inflicted gunshot wounds to mortality is substantial. Personal violence and transportation-related injury are the major causes of death from head injury in each county. Approximately one-half of all transportation-related deaths occurred to occupants of motor vehicles, and one-sixth were the result of motorcycle crashes.

The place of death for all head injury deaths was also determined in the three county survey [16]. Slightly more than 60% of all head injury deaths were immediate deaths and about 10% were reported in emergency rooms. That only one-third survived long enough to receive

Table III. Head injury death rates per 100,000 population and percent causes for Bronx County, N.Y.; Harris County, Tex., and San Diego County, Calif., 1980 [source: Frankowski et al., 16]

Sex	Bronx County	Harris County	San Diego County
Male	42.8	50.2	42.2
Female	11.0	12.6	11.4
Cause			
Transportation-related	21.3%	44.3%	50.2%
Self-inflicted gunshot wound	4.3%	22.8%	19.6%
Other gunshot wound	35.1%	21.1%	8.7%
Falls	18.6%	5.4%	14.7%

inpatient hospital care is a characteristic finding of head injury mortality in the United States [17]. The data suggest that in most cases of fatal head injury the severity of the initial injury is extreme and its course is rapid.

The most consistent characteristic of diffuse brain damage is altered consciousness [1]. The Glasgow Coma Scale [described in paper by *O'Shanick,* this vol.] has been widely adopted by the neurosurgical community as a clinical measure of the severity of a head injury [18] and has been shown to be a discriminating and reliable measure of the continuum of trauma-induced coma [19].

Kraus et al. [13] in the 1981 San Diego County study employed the Glasgow Coma Scale to characterize the initial degree of acute brain injury among all incident cases admitted for hospital care. Patients with a Glasgow Coma Scale of 8 or lower were termed *severe.* Those with a Glasgow Coma Score of 9 through 12, were termed *moderate* if their hospital stay was at least 48 hours *and* one of the following was present: brain surgery or an abnormal CAT scan. All others were termed *mild.*

Annegers et al. [8] in the Olmsted County Study also classified incidence by the severity of injury but defined the degrees of injury by combinations of the type of injuries and duration of LOC or PTA. *Severe* injuries include intracranial hematoma, brain contusion, or LOC for longer than 24 h or PTA of more than 24 h. *Moderate* injuries included either LOC or PTA for 30 min to 24 h, or skull fracture, or both. *Mild* injuries were patients with LOC or PTA of less than 0.5 h

Table IV. Incidence of head injury per 100,000 population by severity of injury as reported in selected studies

Population and year	Mild	Moderate	Severe	Total incidence[1]
San Diego County, 1981 [13]				
acute brain injury	131	15	14	180
Olmsted County, 1965–1974 [8]				
Male	149	69	17	270
Female	71	29	6	116
Evanston, Ill.[2], 1979–1980 [10]	118	20	15	188

[1] Refers to all fatal and nonfatal injuries per 100,000 population.
[2] Evanston whites only.

without skull fracture. *Whitman* [10] in his study of Chicago-area communities employed the severity scale suggested by Annegers.

The severity of incident head injuries reported by selected studies is shown in table IV. Although the severity classification systems used in the studies are not coincident, the systems are broadly comparable. A general feature of table IV is that at least one-half of all incident head injuries may be termed *mild*. *Kraus* et al. [13) report case fatality percents among severe, moderate and mild injuries at 58, 7 and 0.1%, respectively.

The only time trend data on the incidence of head injury comes from the population of Olmsted County [8]. Incidence more than doubled, for both sexes, over the 40-year period, 1935 to 1974. Most of the increase of incidence was in the mild injury category. The increase of incidence occurred primarily within ages 15 through 24 and was associated mainly with increasing numbers of motor vehicle accidents. Moderate, severe, and fatal injury incidences showed little change from 1945 through 1974. The lack of a time trend change in the incidence of fatal injuries is consistent with the earlier noted observation that most fatal head injuries occur too quickly to receive inpatient hospital care. A large number of nonhospital deaths will mask any improved therapeutic survivorship when both hospital and nonhospital deaths are combined in a secular series describing the total incidence of fatal head injury for a population.

Outcome Following Head Injury

Head injury is well known for its potential to cause a wide variety of morbidities. These include neurophysical sequelae, neuropsychological sequelae, psychiatric sequelae, and their interactions which may induce social dysfunction. The articles by *O'Shanick* and by *Hayden and Hart* [this vol.] provide excellent and thorough descriptions of these consequences, their course, and probable etiologies as well as in *Jennett and Teasdale* [1] and *Levin* et al. [20].

The extraordinary range of the sequelae of head injury has necessitated the invention of a global measure of the quality of survival following outcome. The Glasgow Outcome Scale [21] was designed to assess disability following head injury. Its purpose is to quantify the combined effects of specific mental and neurological deficits by general categories of recovery. The Glasgow Outcome Scale recognizes four categories of survival following injury. These categories are the *vegetative state,* describing nonsentient survival; *severe disability,* a conscious but dependent state; *moderate disability,* a category describing individuals disabled but independent; and *good recovery,* a category describing an individual who is able to participate in normal social activities and who can return to work. Although the boundaries between categories of the Glasgow Outcome Scale are not sharp, the scale has been established as a useful guide to the measurement of outcome [22].

The Glasgow Outcome Score was used by *Kraus* et al. [13] to quantify the hospital discharge status of all incident cases of acute brain injury among the 1981 population of San Diego County. Nearly 90% of all incident cases had a *good recovery* on discharge from primary hospital treatment. *Moderate* or *severe* outcomes were reported for 4%, and 0.5% were discharged in a persistent vegetative state; the remaining were fatal injuries. Neurological deficits or limitations were reported at the time of hospital discharge for 5–10% of the patients. Neurologic sequelae included posttraumatic amnesia, paresis, convulsions, or cranial nerve deficits.

The specific extent of cognitive impairment, lack of psychosocial adjustment, and frequency of subjective medical complaints following mild head injury (GCS 13–15 and LOC of less than 20 min) has been a topic of recent interest [23, 24]. *Rimel* et al. [23] in a study of admissions to a regional hospital, suggested that the frequency of neuropsychological and social morbidity may reflect the presence of organic brain damage among patients with mild injuries. This hypothesis is yet to be confirmed or denied by controlled studies of mild injuries.

Risk Factors

Comparison-based epidemiologic research on risk factors associated with head injury is sparse. *Annegers* et al. [8] showed that the incidence rate of head injury increased significantly for second and subsequent head injuries. The increased incidence was independent of gender, but varied with age. The relative risk of a subsequent head injury doubled under age 14, tripled after an injury at ages 15 through 24, and increased fivefold after injuries at age 25 or older. The increase in relative risk of subsequent head injuries among adults was hypothesized to be probably due to behavioral characteristics such as alcohol abuse [8, see also *Reilly* et al., this vol.]. Psychological factors such as family disruption and dissolution, and pre-existing psychiatric disorders have also been suggested as risk factors, but these factors have not been uniformly confirmed by controlled research [20, see also *Leventhal and Midelfort,* this vol.]. Alcohol use shortly before injury is the most commonly cited predisposing factor but its role is complex [1], and surely not unique to head injury.

Risk factors for injury extend well beyond individual susceptibility and behavior. Injury results from a complex set of interactions that involve the person at risk, the agent of energy transmission, and the environment which hosts or supports the specific injury event. The interactions of this triad determine the timing, pathology, and severity of injury, indeed the triad determines whether an injury will actually occur. In an epidemiologic sense, the occurrence of injury is analogous to classic models of infectious disease [27]. Risk factors therefore encompass all of the elements of the chain of events that lead to injury.

Countermeasures are properly directed at elements of the injury triad that will either eliminate or dissipate the injurious nature of a physical energy interchange. Examples of this approach to primary, secondary, and tertiary prevention of unintentional injury are plentiful [25]. The use of window guards to prevent falls among children, design modification of homes to prevent falls among the elderly, and design modifications of motor vehicles, and highway systems to eliminate specific types of vehicle crashes are illustrative of primary prevention.

Secondary prevention is illustrated by helmet use to prevent or markedly reduce motorcycle and pedalcycle injuries, and safety restraining systems for occupants of motor vehicles. Tertiary prevention includes appropriate staging and organization of emergency medical services, primary medical care, and rehabilitation to minimize the effects of injury [27].

Violence, including assault, homicide and suicide is an important cause of head injuries [see also article by *Leventhal and Midelfort,* this vol.]. The literature on risk factors associated with violence is extensive [25–29]. *Waller and Whorton* [30] have suggested, an association within individuals, as yet not explored in great depth. They suggest that deliberate violence and previous unintentional injuries are related events and that both appear closely related to alcohol abuse. Debate on risk factors of violence is plentiful, but solutions and counter-measures at a population level are in short supply [31].

Overview

Accidents, homicide, and suicide are major causes of mortality and morbidity in the United States. Each year these three causes of death claim nearly 160,000 lives [32]. Nearly ⅔ of all fatal injuries are owed to accidents, mostly motor vehicle crashes. The remaining, in near equal numbers, are owed to homicide and suicide. Injury is the major cause of death among the young. It is the leading cause of death for ages 1 through 45, the leading cause of years of productive life lost, a particular threat to the elderly, and the fifth ranked cause of all hospital admissions in the United States [25, 29, 32, 33].

Between ¼ and ⅓ of all fatal injuries in the United States involve a significant intracranial injury. Head injury mortality is predominantly a male affliction. General population head injury mortality is 20–30 head injury deaths per 100,000 population. Most deaths, perhaps up to ⅔, are immediate deaths reflecting the catastrophic nature of most fatal head injuries. In comparison to other western countries, the head injury death rate for the United States is at least twice that reported for England and Scotland, but is similar in both level and demographic correlates to data reported for regions of Australia [34, 35]. The remarkable difference in mortality between the United States and the United Kingdom cannot be accounted for by differences in age structures of the two populations [34]. The explanation likely resides in the distinct patterns of exposure to the risks of severe and fatal head injury of the two populations, and the greater attention of the United Kingdom to programs for the prevention of injury.

Head injuries constitute a substantial but imprecisely known proportion of all injury morbidity in the United States. The difficulties of estimating the total incidence due to all head injuries have been aptly summarized by Jennett [34]:

'It is not possible to state simply how frequently head injuries occur. No universal definition of practical value can be proposed to cover the many minor injuries known only to general practicioners, traffic police, or officials at sporting events and those that are never reported unless complications develop. The actual incidence of head injury is therefore an abstraction. It is, however, reasonable for those concerned with preventing head injuries and planning health services for their care to focus on injuries that lead to death, hospital admission, or attendance at accident departments.'

With this limitation in mind, studies of head injuries in the United States can be interpreted to indicate that the approximate incidence of fatal head injury and nonfatal hospital-treated head injury, with actual or presumed brain involvement, varies from 0.2 to 0.3% per year among large and diverse U.S. populations.

The majority of head injuries appear to be mild, but perhaps up to 30% are serious life-threatening injuries posing significant sequelae to those who survive. Incidence patterns place the young and the elderly at particular risk. Males sustain head injury twice as often as females, reflecting sex difference in the kind, degree, and exposure of males to the hazards of head injury.

The causes of head injuries are obvious. Most result from transportation, fall, or personal violence. Among fatal injuries gunshot injuries are overly abundant; a finding unique to the United States. The appalling feature of the causes of head injury is that for the most part the injuries were preventable. This has not escaped national attention. The reduction of morbidity and mortality from injuries has become one of the national health objectives of the United States for the 1990s [36].

References

1   Jennet, B.; Teasdale, G.: Management of head injuries (Davis, Philadelphia 1981).
2   National Center for Health Statistics: Current estimates from the National Health Interview Survey: United States, 1980. Series 10, No. 139, DDHS Publ. No. (PHS) 82–1567 (Public Health Service, Hyattsville 1981).

3   Caveness, W.: Incidence of craniocerebral trauma in the United States in 1976 with trend from 1970 to 1975; in Thompson, Green. Advances in neurology, vol. 22, pp. 1–3 (Raven Press, New York 1979).

4   Anderson, D.; Kalsbeek, W.; Hartwell, T.: The National Head and Spinal Cord Injury Survey: design and methodology. J. Neurosurg. *53:* S11–S18 (1980).

5   National Center for Health Statistics: Eighth Revision, International Classification of Diseases, Adapted for Use in the United States. PHS Publ. No. 1963 (USGPO, Washington 1967).

6   Kalsbeek, W.; McLaurin, R.; Harris, B.; Miller, J.: The National Head and Spinal Cord Injury Survey: major findings. J. Neurosurg. *53:* S19–S31 (1980).

7   Kraus, J.: Injury to the head and spinal cord: the epidemiological relevance of the literature published from 1960 to 1978. J. Neurosurg. *53:* S3–S10 (1980).

8   Annegers, J.; Grabow, J; Kurland, L.; Laws, E., Jr.: The incidence, causes, and secular trends of head trauma in Olmsted County, Minnesota. Neurology, Minneap. *30:* 912–919 (1980).

9   Cooper, K.; Tabaddor, K.; Hauser, W.; Shulman, K.; Feiner, C.; Factor, P.: The epidemiology of head injury in the Bronx. Neuroepidemiology *2:* 70–88 (1983).

10 Whitman, S.; Coonly-Hoganson, R.; Desai, B.: Comparative head trauma experiences in two socioeconomically different Chicago-area communities: a population study. Am. J. Epidem. *119:* 186–201 (1984).

11 Jagger, J.; Levine, J.; Jane, J.; Rimel, R.: Epidemiologic features of head injury in a predominantly rural population. J. Trauma *24:* 40–44 (1984).

12 Klauber, M.; Barrett-Connor, E.; Marshall, L.; Bowers, S.: The epidemiology of head injury: a prospective study of an entire community-San Diego County, California. Am. J. Epidem. *113:* 500–509 (1978).

13 Kraus, J.; Black, M.; Hessol, N.; Ley, P.; Rokaw, W.; Sullivan, C.; Bowers, S.; Knowlton, S.; Marshall, L.: The incidence of acute brain injury and serious impairment in a defined population. Am. J. Epidem. *119:* 186–201 (1984).

14 Gronwall, D.; Wrighton, P.: Cumulative effect of concussion. Lancet *ii:* 995–997 (1978).

15 National Center for Health Statistics: Multiple causes of death in the United States. Monthly Vital Statistics Report, vol. 32, No. 10, suppl. (2), DHHS Publ. No. (PHS) 84–1120 (Public Health Service, Hyattsville 1984).

16 Frankowski, R.; Klauber, M.; Tabaddor, K.; Marshall L.: Head injury mortality: a comparison of three metropolitan counties (in press, 1985).

17 Frankowski, R.; Annegers, J.; Whitman, S.: The descriptive epidemiology of head trauma in the United States; in Becker, Povlishock, Status report in central nervous system trauma, NINCDS (in press, 1985).

18 Teasdale, A.; Jennett, B.: Assessment of coma and impaired consciousness; a practical scale. Lancet *ii:* 81–84 (1974).

19 Teasdale, G.; Knill-Jones, R.; Van der Sande, J.: Observer variability in assessing impaired consciousness and coma. J. Neurol. Neurosurg. Psychiat. *41:* 603–610 (1978).

20 Levin H.; Benton A.; Grossman, R.: Neurobehavioral consequences of closed head injury (Oxford University Press, Oxford 1982).

21 Jennett B.; Bond, M.: Assessment of outcome after severe brain damage. Lancet *i:* 480–487 (1975).

22 Mass, A.; Braakman, R.; Schouten, H.; Minderhoud, J.; Van Zomeren, A.,: Agreement between physicians on assessment of outcome following severe head injury. J. Neurosurg. *58:* 321–325 (1985).

23 Rimel, R.; Giordani, B.; Barth, J.; Boll, T.; Jane, J.: Diability caused by minor head injury. Neurosurgery *9:* 221–227 (1981).

24 Barth, J.; Macciocchi, S.; Giordani, B.; Rimel, R.; Jane, J.; Boll, T: Neuropsychological sequelae of minor head injury. Neurosurgery *13* 529–533 (1983).

25 Waller, J.: Injury control; a guide to the causes and prevention of trauma (Heath, Lexington 1985).

26 Flamm, E.; Demopoulaus, H.; Seligman, M.; Tomasula, J.; DeCrescito, V.; Ransohoff, J.: Ethanol potentiation of central nervous system trauma. J. Neurosurg. *46:* 328–335 (1977).

27 Haddon, W., Jr.: Advances in the epidemiology of injuries as a basis for public policy. Publ. Hlth Rep. *95:* 411–421 (1980).

28 Baker, S.; O'Neill, B.; Karpf, R.: The injury fact book (Lexington Books, Lexington 1984).

29 Robertson, L.: Injuries; causes control strategies, and public policy (Heath, Lexington 1983).

30 Waller, J.; Whorton, E.: Unintentional shootings, highway crashes, and acts of violence: a behavioral paradigm. Accident Anal. Prevent. *5:* 351–356 (1973).

31 Whitman, S; McKnight, J.: Ideology and injury prevention. Int. J. Hlth Serv. *15:* 35–46 (1985).

32 National Center for Health Statistics: Advance report, final mortality statistics, 1982. Monthly Vital Statistics Report, vol. 33, No. 9, suppl., DHHS Publ. No. (PHS) 85–1120 (Public Health Service, Hyattsville 1984).

33 National Center for Health Statistics: Inpatient utilization of shortstay hospitals by diagnosis: United States, 1980. Series 13, No. 74, DDHS Publ. No. (PHS) 83–1735 (Public Health Service, Hyattsville 9183).

34 Jennett, B.; MacMillian, R.: Epidemiology of head injuries. Br. med. J. *282:* 101–104 (1981).

35 McEwin, R.: Head injuries in New South Wales: incidence; in Dinning, Connelley, Proceedings of a National Symposium: head injuries, a preventable epidemic, Sydney 1981. Head injuries, an integrated approach, pp. 9–14 (Wiley, Brisbane 1981).

36 Davis, H., Jr.; Schletty, A.; Ing, R.; Weisman, R.: The 1990 objectives for the nation for injury prevention: a progress review. Publ. Hlth Rep. *99:* 10–24 (1984).

Ralph F. Frankowski, PhD, The University of Texas, School of Public Health, P.O. Box 20186, Houston, TX 77225 (USA)

Adv. psychosom. Med., vol. 16, pp. 173–193 (Karger, Basel 1986)

Neuropsychiatric Complications in Head Injury

Gregory J. O'Shanick

Medical Psychiatry Service, Medical College of Virginia, Richmond, Va., USA

Neuropsychiatric Sequela of Head Trauma

'A good outcome to the doctor may be a disaster to the patient and family.'

Bryan Jennett

Sophisticated, rapid neurosurgical intervention has greatly increased the survival rate of previously fatal head trauma. As a result of this, survivors and their families now face a constellation of sequellae including significant morbidity in the personal, social, and economic spheres. Current literature provides an exhaustive consideration of the acute neurosurgical management [1] and the various rehabilitation avenues available for these complex and multiply-impaired individuals [2, 3]. Yet, the neuropsychiatric sequellae are frequently neglected in the overall treatment program of these patients. Clinicians treating patients with histories of head trauma must be aware of the complex interaction of previous personality style, severity of traumatic injury, co-existing medical-surgical factors, and environmental supports. These components must be considered to maximize psychosocial recovery and forestall disastrous personal consequences for the patient despite excellent 'neurosurgical recovery'.

General Considerations

Epidemiologic characterization of head trauma patients has been biased towards the more severely injured. Hospital-based statistics and mortality reviews suggest an incidence of 200/100,000 population per year [4] which is equivalent to the incidence of cerebrovascular accidents (CVA) [5]. However, unlike CVA, head trauma is principally a 'disease' of young adult males [6]. Peak incidence is between the ages of 15 and 25 with males outnumbering females by 4 to 1. Another peak is evident in the geriatric population when men are twice as likely to experience head trauma. With a peak incidence in an age group in the initial stages of occupational or scholastic productivity, the economic impact of this loss is staggering. A 1979 study [7] suggests the annual economic impact of these patient's loss to society to be approximately $2 billion!

Substance abuse has a robust association in the genesis of head trauma. Studies note an average of 32% [8] of head trauma patients to be intoxicated at admission. Gender differences exist within these statistics such that 29% of the men and 11% of the women have evidence of past substance abuse [9]. Patients seen at a major trauma center in Houston, Tex., studied by the author had a higher rate of both ethanol abuse (36%) and other substance abuse (21%) [10]. The typical scenario is one in which drunk driving young men hit drunk old pedestrians resulting in head trauma to both.

The organic substrate for behavioral and physical sequelae has been studied extensively. Experimental models [11] and clinical correlations of computerized tomography (CT) [12, 13], electrophysiologic changes [14, 15], neurotransmitter [16–19], and autopsy [20, 21] findings have improved understanding of the pathophysiology of this condition.

Holbourn [22] utilized a gelatin 'brain' in a wax 'skull' to demonstrate the 'shear-strain' effect which resulted from sudden rotational forces similar to those incurred in head injury. The anterior temporal lobe region showed the most prominent strain, although frontal regions were also affected. By replacing monkey calvaria with transparent covers, *Pudenz* and *Sheldon* [23] noted the swirling motion after impact of the brain and found these motions to be most prominent when the head was not restricted in movement. These studies lent support to the clinical correlative data noting coup and contre coup lesions in frontal and anterior temporal regions [24].

Shear-strain effects also correlate with the diffuse neuronal damage found in postmortem studies. Autopsy data from patients surviving for one year resulted in *Strich's* [25] observation that impact caused primary neuronal damage followed by more diffuse white matter degeneration. (The importance of loss of cell membrane integrity has been noted and thought to be secondary to alterations in sodium and potassium permeability resulting in edema and neuronal drop out [26]. Autopsy changes, consistent with microscopic white matter degeneration, have been noted in frontal and temporal regions, the corpus callosum, and the hypothalamus [27]. The role of shear-strain in the genesis of these changes is now accepted. As these changes are microscopic in nature, computerized tomographic (CT) findings in these patients are often negligible.

Electroencephalographic changes are common in patients after head trauma and show a progression of changes in dominant frequency. Diffuse slowing is seen in the immediate post-traumatic period with gradual return to normal beta and alpha frequencies as the injury resolves [28]. Other changes may evolve if abstinence syndromes emerge or if other metabolic derangements exist. Medication artifact may also be detected and further confuse the interpretation of the EEG in head trauma patients. In those who develop post-traumatic epilepsy, focal activity is noted to persist. Algorhythms for predicting the likelihood of epilepsy have been developed involving assessment of the presence of dural tears, hemorrhage into the cerebrospinal fluid, and parenchymal damage [29].

Endocrine changes after head trauma have been the subject of study especially in relation to the shear-strain effect on the hypothalamus and the pituitary stalk [30]. Hormonal studies have focused principally on comatose individuals and have concluded that disruption of all adrenal, thyroid, growth, and gonadic hormones can occur [31–33]. The syndrome of diabetes insipidus also is well studied in these patients and mandates urgent medical attenuation. One difficulty in assessing endocrine function has been failure to address the effects of routine anticonvulsant treatment in these conditions on provocative tests of pituitary function and pituitary reserves and also with protein binding of the active hormone. Further endocrine evaluation is required in those patients who do not experience coma, to better elucidate the significance of these changes alone.

Neurotransmitter studies in head trauma patients have focused on the metabolites of dopamine (i.e. homovanillic acid, HVA), and serotonin (i.e. 5-hydroxy-indole acetic acid, 5HIAA). Since 1975, only 5 such investigations have been published with none focused on the behavioral changes associated with neurotransmitter changes. In general, HVA is elevated early in diffuse damage [17] when associated with elevated intracranial pressure and gradually subsides as a chronic, demented state evolves [16, 18]. An initial elevation of 5HIAA has been noted in patients with diffuse damage [17]; however, more focal frontotemporal trauma has been associated with lower 5HIAA levels [19]. Other investigators note no change in 5HIAA levels over time regardless of clinical state [16]. Certainly, more rigorous investigation is required to evaluate the behavioral consequences of these fluctuations.

Efforts to track the evolution of symptoms in head trauma have characteristically focused on anterograde amnesia, i.e. memory loss for events subsequent to the traumatic event, a consistent finding in head injury. Termed 'post-traumatic amnesia' (PTA) in 1946 by *Russell and Nathan* [34], the duration of this symptom is variable, but generally correlates with long-term prognosis [35]. Retrograde amnesia, i.e. for events prior to the trauma, is also observed clinically; however, the utility of the resolution of this phenomenon has not been established vis-à-vis outcome.

Although rich in descriptive language and clinical profiles, early studies of head trauma lacked uniformity of evaluative instruments to permit rigorous comparisons [36–38]. Three such clinical ratings are now routinely accepted and enable more distinctive categorization of patients for both treatment and outcome analysis.

Teasdale and Jennett [39] developed the Glasgow Coma Scale (GCS) to assess the initial severity of the event (table I). By measuring three clinical features of the head-injured patient (eye movement, motor response, and verbal response), division of the clinical syndrome of head trauma into mild (≥ 13), moderate (9–12), and severe (≤ 8) was possible and permitted more valid comparisons of similarly compromised patients. Widely used in the United States, Great Britain and Australia, the GCS holds generally good interrater reliability and clinical correlation.

To assess cognition after head trauma, Levin developed the Galveston Orientation and Amnesia Test (GOAT) for use in the subacute stage of recovery [40]. By measuring orientation to person, place, and time as well as historical events before and after the accident, the GOAT provides a relatively uniform measure of the period of post-traumatic amnesia. GOAT scores have been used in conjunction with GCS and bear a strong relationship to these acute ratings. The daily

Table I. Glasgow Coma Scale

Eye opening
    1 None (not due to facial edema)
    2 To pain (stimulation to chest/limbs)
    3 To speech (nonspecific response)
    4 Spontaneous

Motor response to pain stimulus or command
    1 No response (flaccid)
    2 Extension ('decerebrate')
    3 Abnormal flexion ('decorticate')
    4 Withdrawal (normal flexor response)
    5 Localizes pain (purposeful movement)
    6 Obeys commands

Verbal response
    1 None
    2 Incomprehensible (moans)
    3 Inappropriate ('loose associations')
    4 Confused ('delirious')
    5 Oriented fully

GCS = E + M + V (3–15).

---

monitoring of patient improvement on the GOAT also encourages the mandatory orientation exercises for these patients. Scores of 70–75% on the GOAT are by convention held to reflect the end of PTA and the point at which more active information retrieval is possible.

The Brief Psychiatric Rating Scale (BPRS) was initially developed as a rapid assessment technique for psychiatric characteristics (tension, emotional withdrawal, mannerisms/posturing, motor retardation, uncooperativeness) and verbal production (conceptual disorganization, unusual thought content, anxiety, guilt, grandiosity, depressive mood, hostility, somatic concern, hallucinatory behavior, suspiciousness, blunted affect). Use of the BPRS with head trauma patients has correlated emotional isolation, blunted affect, excitability, and conceptual disorganization with electroencephalographic (EEG) and computerized tomographic (CT) abnormalities [42]. The serial performance of BPRS permits longitudinal assessment of behavioral change in an objective, replicable manner.

Table II. Neuropsychiatric evaluation after head injury

Historical data (from patient and reliable third parties)
    Present history (including Glasgow Coma Score)
    Type of injury (deceleration, motor vehicle, etc.)
    History of previous head injury
    Psychiatric history (patient and family)
    Medical history (recent, past, ROSS, allergies)
    Habits (ethanol, illicit drugs, medications, work, social, nutritional)
    Current therapies

Objective data
    Mental status examination (extensive cognitive, aphasia, and affective focus)
    GCS, GOAT, BPRS
    Vital signs
    Physical examination (with complete neurological examination)

Laboratory evaluation
    Blood alcohol level
    Drug screen
    Complete blood count
    Urinalysis
    Electrolytes
    VDRL
    Blood chemistry (hepatic, renal, etc.)
    Nutritional parameters (B_{12}, Folate, Mg, Zn, Cu)
    Endocrine parameters (thyroid function tests, plasma cortisol, prolactin level,
        FSH/LH, growth hormone
    Arterial blood gases (carbon monoxide)

Radiographic/Electrophysiologic Evaluation
    Chest X-ray
    Electroencephalogram (EEG) with nasopharyngeal leads
    Evoked potentials (brain stem auditory evoked)
    Computer assisted tomography (with and without contrast)
    Nuclear magnetic resonance (NMR)

The complex physiologic changes which occur subsequent to head trauma must be considered in the development of any behavioral disturbance in these patients. Neuropsychiatric evaluation mandates the assessment of multiple organic factors which are all well known to induce behavioral symptomatology [43, 44]. In addition to routine hematology and blood chemistry studies, evaluation of endocrine, electrophysiologic, and nutritional parameters along with assessment of illicit substances which might produce abstinence syndromes (table II) are necessary.

Clinical Syndromes

Behavioral change that evolves after head trauma can be conceptualized along the same time continuum noted above. The psychosocial symptoms can be managed by utilizing a matrix as shown in table III. This format provides accurate and rapid assessment for psychosocial problems which may evolve at any point in the recovery process and suggests interventions (biologic, psychologic, or social) at the level of the patient, his family, and the staff caring for him.

Acute Phase

The acute phase of head trauma is defined by loss of consciousness (i.e. coma). While this period may be so brief in duration as to be clinically nondetectable, in other cases it may involve a more protracted course. The mechanism involved in coma is believed to relate to brain stem dysfunction, specifically disruption of those ascending cholinergic fibers known as the 'ascending reticular activating system' [45]. Comatose patients require high level, meticulous supportive nursing care and should also receive some level of sensory stimulation daily. A tendency towards treating comatose patients as inanimate objects should be avoided in favor of an interactive style which orients the patient to his surroundings and situation in a consistent, concise manner.

Psychosocial intervention at this stage is directed primarily at family members who may be in the early stages of grief and adaptation to the social role changes that occur after catastrophic illness [46]. In severe situations, family members may require brief treatment (1–2 weeks) with anxiolytic medications to stabilize sleep patterns and permit them to assume their new responsibilities in a composed fashion. The use of family support groups as a means of addressing the informational and ventilatory needs of families is a time-efficient format for intervention at this stage. Assisting families to better organize their interfacing with the medical care team contributes greatly to the expeditious care of the patient and eases the time burden of the treating physician. Families must also be aided in obtaining legal guardianship (when necessary) to provide for competent longitudinal care for the patient as he recovers.

In the course of treating comatose patients, staff members may become increasingly less empathic and dehumanize the patient. These developments should alert one to the evolution of a staff 'burn-out' syndrome or an overidentification with the patient or his family. Staff members on active head trauma units may require either formal or informal group meetings to permit the expression of frustration, grief, and anger which is a normal aspect of caring for these difficult (and emotionally unresponsive) patients and their families [47].

Subacute Phase

Upon emerging from coma, the patient enters a period of marked disorientation and distortion of perceptial modalities. This post-traumatic amnestic (PTA) phase is similar in symptomatology to delirium from other causes and is presumably due to diffuse neuronal dysfunction after the traumatic event [48]. Delirium can be aggravated by other factors including abstinence syndromes, malnutrition, hypoxia, metabolic and electrolytic disturbances, anemia, and environmental changes [49].

Attentional deficits may exist singularly or in combination with disruption of sleep-wake cycles. Patients often become agitated or combative at the slightest provocation. They may frequently misinterpret external stimuli (i.e. illusions) or experience true hallucinatory phenomenon (visual, tactile, auditory, or olfactory in nature). Such episodes are most typically observed to occur at transition points in the patient's daily routine, including true hypnogogic (at sleep) or hypnopompic (on awakening) phenomenon.

Treatment of the PTA-delirium phenomenon should address multiple intervention strategies. Abstinence syndromes should be anticipated and treated vigorously [50]. Ethanol withdrawal, while typically evolving 71–96 h after the last drink, may be delayed by the use of anesthetic agents which have cross-tolerance properties. Benzodiazepine abstinence phenomenon may occur at therapeutic doses prescribed by out-patient physicians and may present as late as four weeks after the last dose [51]. For an in-depth review of these disorders and their treatment, the reader is referred to *Khantzian and McKenna's* [52] article.

Malnutrition is an often overlooked complication of this phase [1]. Age, social class, and substance abuse may render these patients at risk pre-morbidly and assessment of thiamine, folate, and B_{12} levels is essential [53]. Protracted coma or PTA may preclude adequate nutrition and evaluation of levels of magnesium, copper, and zinc is mandated to reduce potential deficiencies of these trace elements [54].

Physiologic disturbance may also worsen PTA. Anemia, with or without hypoxemia, needs to be corrected. Electrolytic disturbances such as hyponatremia or hyperkalemia demand correction as do hepatic and renal dysfunction with accompanying azotemia and hyperammonemia.

Psychopharmacologic intervention is aimed at rapid neuroleptization of these patients with low dose, high potency neuroleptics such as haloperidol or fluphenazine. Neuroleptics should be given intravenously to permit the most rapid lysis of symptoms [55]. Doses should be scheduled to coincide with changes in the patient's environment: e.g. at shift change, at bedtime, prior to dressing changes. Evidence now exists suggesting a negative effect of neuroleptics on the rehabilitation process [56]. Use of such agents should be carefully weighed against other physical means of controlling agitation and combativeness. Physical restraint may be preferable and should be implemented using *leather* restraints which consistently and securely discourage activity. Severe cases may require the use of both neuroleptics and physical restraint. In these instances, a more sedating neuroleptic (e.g. droperidol, 6–12 mg i.v. or i.m.) may more rapidly diminish agitation and sedate the patient effectively at night [59]. The use of benzodiazepines or barbiturates to control these patients is to be discouraged. Both classes of psychotropics are prone to induce an increase in agitation and a disinhibition of aggressive behavior [58].

Psychological intervention during the period of PTA is directed towards assisting the patient's return of informational processing. At least on a daily basis, patients should be queried regarding their surroundings, the date, the nature of their illness, and their memory of events prior to the accident. The use of the GOAT provides a standardized test for staff and family to use in this process [40]. Family members are encouraged to bring objects and memorabilia from home to stimulate the patient's interest in his hospital environment and create a more familiar, secure milieu.

Continuous sensory stimulation may assist some patients in their re-orientation to the environment. Calendars and clocks should be routinely present and night lights should be used. Use of radio and television as orienting tools needs to be measured against the excess stimulation of such media to some acutely agitated individuals.

Some individuals in the PTA phase do not experience profound agitation and combativeness. Frequently, disruption in sleep-wake cycle is the sole manifestation of this phase from a behavioral perspective. Initial interventions directed towards getting the patient out of his room and into well-traveled corridors may increase daytime arousal; however, pharmacologic assistance may be required to initiate sleep. As sleep initiation has been associated with serotonin activity [59], agents which potentiate this neurotransmitter are preferred. Trazodone [60] and amitriptyline [61], both of which are antidepressants, inhibit serotonin re-uptake at the synapse and may be of benefit in these patients. The anticholinergic properties of amitriptyline may elicit objectionable side effects in patients at therapeutic doses (150 mg/day) and may complicate compliance.

As the period of PTA resolves, patients may develop sleep disturbance secondary to having intrusive, vivid dreams of the traumatic event. This development, in association with affective blunting, increased autonomic arousal and hyperattentiveness to external stimuli, may herald the onset of a post-traumatic stress disorder [62]. Intervention is directed at decreasing intrusive thoughts or dreams by using an antidepressant (e.g. imipramine) [63] and decreasing general arousal responses by using relaxation training or biofeedback techniques.

Specific problems emerge for the patient's family during the PTA phase. While most greet the transition from coma to some degree of consciousness with great hope and expectation, often unrealistic and premature demands are placed upon the patient which far exceed his ability. The family's joy at a loved ones 'survival' may be hastily squelched in the face of a combative, agitated, confabulating 'stranger'. In addition to the demands these patients place upon the financial resources of their families, families are also engaged by staff to actively interface with the patient and assist with re-orienting exercises [40].

The mourning and adaptation to stress, which may have proceeded uneventfully for the family while the patient was comatose, must now reorganize to include a more vivid reminder of the loss. While the patient most often externally appears the same, his behavior and interpersonal style are foreign. Families report that this consistent reminder of their loss precludes any successful resolution of their mourning.

In situations where other individuals have been involved in the accident and died, family members are faced with the difficult task of fielding questions from the recovering patient and responding to the emotions generated. Massive support is required to aid the family in their re-examination of their own mourning as they 'break the news' to the patient [46].

While staff in the acute care setting can function to some extent in an emotionally detached fashion, the emotional demands of caring for patients in the PTA phase vary greatly. A flexible response is critical to the management of these patients whose needs vary from total supportive care to strict limitsetting and behavioral shaping to empathic management of their mourning process often within the same 8-hour shift! Staff morale and emotional health is of paramount importance for the active head trauma unit to function smoothly. Scheduling and patient assignments should be made fairly. Those individuals demonstrating proficiency and comfort with certain phase-specific events should be used as 'specialists' and as resources for other staff who have patients displaying a certain behavior. Consistent care is essential for the patient's optimal recovery. Care plans and treatment strategies should be coordinated in planning conferences to assure 24-hour consistency.

A common complication for the family, staff, and physician during the PTA phase is the confusion arising from the patient's confabulation. This is especially frequent in patients with bifrontal injuries [64]. In their earnest desire to interact with their environment, patients may create plausible, yet inconsistent, stories. Open communication among families, staff, and doctors can circumvent premature and disastrous tacit acceptance of these productions. Collateral validation of all patient reports and historical information is mandatory in the PTA phase. Legal guardianship may be required to preclude the patient's inadvertent discharge at this point.

Table III. Clinical syndromes – Focus of intervention

	Patient	Family	Staff
Acute phase	*B*	B	B
	P	*P*	*P*
	S	S	S
Subacute phase	*B*	B	B
	P	P	P
	S	S	S
Chronic phase	*B*	B	B
	P	P	P
	S	S	S

B = Biological; P = psychological; S = social.

Chronic Phase

The beginning of the chronic phase is heralded by resolution of PTA. At this point, the patient is attempting to integrate previous events and to reestablish memory registration and retrieval for the PTA period. Improvement is observed on measures of orientation, immediate recall, short term memory, and anterograde amnesia. Higher level conceptual skills (e.g. abstraction, judgement, insight) continue to show some degree of impairment. Several neuropsychiatric syndromes may present at this point and require thorough evaluation and directive intervention (table III).

Site-specific syndromes may develop where discrete lesions have occurred in the central nervous system [65]. Frontotemporal lesions may induce attentional deficits which preclude effective engagement in the rehabilitation process. White matter degeneration in the corpus collosum results in interhemispheric disconnection syndromes which may mimic the affective blunting seen in major affective disorders [6]. Disruption of the hypothalamic interconnection with the pituitary may produce various endocrinopathies many of which present as mood changes [67]. Lesions in the parietal region, albeit infrequent in closed head injury, result in 'hemi-neglect' phenomenon whereby the individual literally 'forgets' the contralateral side of his body exists [68]. Auditory function may be significantly impaired as a result of shearing of the auditory nerve (CN VIII) resulting in unilateral or bilateral dysfunction [69]. Patients in this phase require a thorough re-evaluation of their organic status prior to entry into comprehensive rehabilitation programs. (Brain stem lesions generally result in persistence of the comatose state (e.g. persistent vegetative state) and require total supportive care rather than rehabilitation.)

Persistent and fixed changes in energy, attentiveness, interpersonal engagement, and periodic irritability may occur and are diagnosed as organic personality syndromes [70]. In cases of persistent episodic extreme irritability or agitation, intermittent explosive disorder may be diagnosed [71]. Failure to recall these outbursts or confabulation by the patient necessitates the separate interviewing of family members to ascertain the presence of these behaviors. This collateral information is also important as frequently these patients have paranoid features which preclude their total candidness with the clinician.

Treatment of these personality syndromes must consider the presumed biologic basis of these phenomena as well as the psychological and social ramifications. Animal and human studies suggest that periodic irritability may indicate electrophysiologic or neurochemical abnormalities of the limbic system [72]. Paroxysmal events may be detected on repeated electroencephalography using sleep deprivation, nasopharyngeal or sphenoidal leads, and various provocative maneuvers (photic driving, overventilation); however, clinical evidence may be the sole positive finding. Management with anticovulsants [73, 74] (diphenylhydantoin, carbamazepine) or beta-adrenergic antagonists (propranolol) [75] may need to be initiated in the face of 'normal' studies. Controversy exists regarding the use of GABA agonists such as benzodiazepines as they may worsen dyscontrol [58]. Studies with lithium have noted some improvement in these patients especially those with combined affective or behavioral disorders [76]. As some evidence exists of serotonin deficit and noradrenergic excess in episodic dyscontrol syndrome [77], the use of antidepressants which preferentially block serotonin re-uptake (e.g. amitriptyline and trazodone) can be helpful. Treatment with stimulants (dextroamphetamine, methylphenidate) has been reported to be effective [78]; however, the abuse potential is quite high in all but well-supervised settings. The general use of neuroleptics at this stage is not encouraged. Evidence exists suggesting impairment of cognitive retraining during exposure to these agents which block not only dopamine receptors, but all catecholamine receptors [56]. Controversy also exists regarding their ability to lower seizure threshold and further expose the patient to the risk of other paroxysmal disturbance [79].

Affective disturbance has been reported to occur in up to 60% of individuals after head trauma [80]. While mourning the loss of the idealized self certainly plays a role in this phenomenon, changes which occur post-head injury in biogenic amines may define a biologically-mediated depressive disorder or more specifically an organic affective syndrome as per DSM-III [81]. Both agitated and retarded psycho-motor activity can be observed [82]. Cognitive clouding secondary to the depressive episode (i.e. pseudodementia) may worsen the patient's performance in the rehabilitation setting.

Treatment of affective disorders post-head injury requires consideration of the multiple receptor sites influenced by antidepressants [61]. Use of secondary amine tricyclics allows monitoring of plasma levels with a defined 'therapeutic window' and permits a somewhat more objective determination of therapeutic dose [83, 84]. Published literature is sparse regarding the treatment of these secondary depressions; however, a study has recently been described showing therapeutic response to nortriptyline in a group of patients who became depressed after cerebrovascular accident [85]. The anticholinergic properties of antidepressant agents may negatively influence cognition and precipitate delirium in some instances. Antidepressants with low anticholinergic properties are trazodone [86] and desipramine [61]. Trazodone, a nontricyclic antidepressant, functions primarily by blocking serotonin re-uptake at the presynaptic level [60]. Desipramine, a secondary amine tricyclic, blocks norepinephrine re-uptake and has a therapeutic window. Trazodone has generally proven to be more sedating than desipramine.

Cognitive dysfunction after head trauma has been well described in the literature for the past 130 years. Recent advances in cognitive retraining have achieved good results, but are beyond the scope of this chapter to consider. Efforts to maximize an individual's success at cognitive rehabilitation requires consideration of several parameters aside from primary neuronal damage and loss. At this time, only anecdotal evidence exists which advocates the use of cholinergic potentiating drugs in cognitive therapy after head trauma [87]. Further well-controlled studies are necessary before any conclusions can be drawn.

Diminished concentration may result from profound depression or impaired perception of the stimulus at hand. Perceptual distortion may result from misinterpretation of the stimulus or failure to acknowledge the stimulus as well as interference by hallucinatory activity. Attention can be disrupted by similar events and also by enhanced sensitivity (or decreased filtering) to coincident stimuli. This can occur due to front-otemporal trauma or post-traumatic stress disorder. Emotional incontinence, as seen in pseudobulbar palsy can adversely impact upon cognitive rehabilitation by disrupting attention and concentration. All these processes should be vigorously treated in concurrence with cognitive therapy [2, 3].

Family disturbances during the chronic phase have been clearly documented in the literature. *Brooks and McKinlay* [88], in their follow-up of 55 families found hypersexuality, aggression, calculated viciousness, apathy, childish behavior, and incontinence to be the most frequently distressing behaviors to family members. *Rosenbaum and Najenson* [89] after 1 year noted a high incidence of depressive disorders among wives of head injured patients. Other families continue to actively deny the severity of cognitive and psychosocial deficit evidenced by the patient. The generalized social isolation of the patient after head injury also inflicts significant social isolation upon the family [90]. Loss of previous support systems is commonly reported.

Certainly, appropriate intervention is required for those family members displaying major affective disorders and antidepressants may be indicated. Psychotherapeutic endeavors should include not only ample ventilation and expression of anger and resentment, but also encouragement to involve the family in various self-help organizations. These provide a cohort of families with similar problems while channeling anger into a socially productive area (e.g. MADD). Family members may require overt permission to take 'vacations' from the patient and hospital respite or day care may be required for brief intervals. Family therapy may or may not be essential.

Staff problems which arise in the chronic phase generally relate less to the type of patient than to the episodic discouragement encountered with specific emotionally draining patients [91]. These patients may be identified by their age, incredible history, or pre-existent psychopathology. Previous diagnosis of borderline personality disorder in a head trauma patient or his family may result in division of the staff into 'good' and 'bad' factions [92]. Such polarities need to be confronted immediately and the staff united to optimize the rehabilitation of the patient. Abundant references are available regarding the importance of supportive groups for staff and more active participation by staff members in the decision making process during rehabilitation. The more responsibility the staff has for the treatment recommendations, the less victimized they feel in a crisis.

Conclusion

The event of head injury is one which epitomizes the complex interaction of biologic, psychologic, and social factors for the patient, his family, the staff caring for him, and for society as a whole. While advances in emergency management have dramatically improved acute survival, treatment options for those with chronic impairment is limited except in those few centers where active research and educational missions have fostered comprehensive rehabilitation programs. In a period of fiscal constraint and cost-containment, efforts to widen the services available to these individuals are difficult at best. Well-planned and controlled studies need to be performed which identify not only cost-effective comprehensive rehabilitation methods, but also more definitive studies on natural history and spontaneous recovery in these groups. Preventive measures such as mandatory child-restraint laws, helmet laws for motorcyclists, and more stringent drunk-driving laws will also impact upon those vectors which precede these costly tragedies.

References

1   Jennett, B.; Teasdale, G.: Management of head injuries (Davis, Philadelphia 1981).
2   Goldstein, G.; Ruthven, L.: Rehabilitation of the brain-damaged adult (Plenum Press, New York 1983).
3   Rosenthal, M.; Griffith E.; Bond, M.; Miller, J.: Rehabilitation of the head injured adult (Davis, Philadelphia 1983).
4   Kalsbeck, W.; McLaurin, R.; Harris, B.; Miller, J.: The national head and spinal cord injury survey: major findings. J. Neurosurg. *53:* 519–531 (1980).
5   Kurtze, J.; Kurtland, L.: The epidemiology of neurologic disease; in Baker, Baker, Clinical neurology, No. 3 (Harper & Row, Hagerstown 1973).
6   Annegers, J.; Grabow, J.; Kurtland, L.; Laws, E.: The incidence, causes, and secular

trends of head trauma in Olmstead County, Minnesota. Neurology, Minneap. *30:* 912–919 (1980).

7   Leigh, D.: Psychiatric aspects of head injury. Psychiat. Dig. *40:* 21–33 (1979).

8   Edna, T.: Alcohol influence and head injury. Acta chir. scand. *148:* 209–212 (1982).

9   Field, J.: Epidemiology of head injury in England and Wales: with particular application to rehabilitation. Leicester (Printed for HM Stationary Office by Willson's, London 1976).

10 O'Shanick, G.; Scott, R.; Peterson, L.: Psychiatric referral after head trauma. Psychiat. Med. *2:* 131–137 (1984).

11 Denny-Brown, D.; Russel, W.: Experimental cerebral concussion. Parts II and III. Brain *64:* 7–164 (1941).

12 Clifton, G.; Grossman, R.; Makela, M.; Miner, M.; Handel, S.; Sadhu, V.: Neurological course and correlated computerized tomography findings after severe closed head injury. J. Neurosurg. *52:* 611–624 (1980).

13 Dongen, K. van; Braakman, R.: Late computed tomography in survivors of severe head injury. Neurosurgey *7:* 14–22 (1980).

14 Greenberg, R.; Mayer, D.; Becker, D.; Miller, J.: Evaluation of brain function in severe human head trauma with multimodality evoked potentials. I. Evoked brain-injury potentials, methods, and analysis. J. Neurosurg. *47:* 150–162 (1977).

15 Greenberg, R.; Becker, D.; Miller, J.; Mayer, D.: Evaluation of brain function in severe human head trauma with multimodality evoked potentials. II. Localization of brain dysfunction and correlation with post-traumatic neurological conditions. J. Neurosurg. *47:* 163–177 (1977).

16 Bareggi, S.; Porta, M.; Selenati, A.; Assael, B.; Calderini, G.; Collice, M.; Rossanda, M.; Morselli, P.: Homovanillic acid and 5-hydroxyindole-acetic acid in the CSF of patients after a severe head injury, I. Lumbar CSF concentration in chronic brain post-traumatic syndromes. Eur. Neurol. *13:* 528–544 (1975).

17 Porta, M.; Bareggi S.; Collice, M.; Assael, B.; Selenati, A.; Calderini, G.; Rossanda, M.; Morselli, P.: Homovanillic acid and 5-hydroxyindole-acetic acid in the CSF of patients after a severe head injury. II. Ventricular CSF concentrations in acute brain post-traumatic syndromes. Eur. Neurol. *13:* 545–554 (1975).

18 Vecht, C.; van Woerkom, T.; Teelken, A.; Minderhoud, J.: Homovanillic acid and 5-hydroxyindoleacetic acid cerebrospinal fluid levels: a study with and without probenecid administration of their relationship to the state of consciousness after head injury. Achs Neurol. *32:* 792–797 (1975).

19 Woerkom, T. van; Teelken, A.; Minderhoud, J.: Difference in neurotransmitter metabolism in frontotemporal-lobe contusion and diffuse cerebral contusion. Landet *i:* 812–813 (1977).

20 Adams, J.; Mitchell, D.; Graham, D.; Doyle, D.: Diffuse Brain damage of immediate impact type: its relationship to 'primary brain-stem damage' in head injury. Brain *100:* 489–502 (1977).

21 Letcher, F.; Corrao, P.; Ommaya, A.: Head injury in the champanzee. II. Spontaneous and evoked epidural potentials as indices of injury severity. J. Neurosurg. *39:* 167–177 (1973).

22 Holbourn, A.: Mechanics of head injury. Lancet *ii:* 438–441 (1943).

23 Pudenz, R.; Sheldon, C.: The lucite calvarium – a method for direct observation of the brain. II. Cranial trauma and brain movement. J. Neurosurg. *3:* 487–505 (1946).

24 Ommaya, A.; Grubb, R.; Naumann, R.: Coup and contre-coup injury: observations on the mechanics of visible brain injuries in the rhesus monkey. J. Neurosurg. *35:* 503–516 (1971).

25 Strich, S.: Diffuse degeneration of the cerebral white matter in severe dementia following head injury. J. Neurol. Neurosurg. Psychiat. *19:* 163–185 (1956).

26 Kimelberg, H.; Bourke, R.; Stieg, P.; Barron, K.; Hirata, H.; Pelton, E.; Nelson, L.: Swelling of astroglia after injury to the central nervous system: mechanisms and consequences; in Grossman, Gildenberg, Head injury: basic and clinical aspects, pp. 31–44 (Raven Press, New York 1982).

27 Brooks, D.; Aughton, M.; Bond, M.; Jones, P.; Rizvi, S.: Cognitive sequelae in relationship to early indices of severity of brain damage after severe blunt head injury. J. Neurol. Neurosurg, Psyhciat. *43:* 529–534 (1980).

28 Dawson, R.; Webster, J.; Gurojian, E.: Serial electroencephalography in acute head injuries. J. Neurosurg. *8:* 613–630 (1951).

29 Feeney, D.; Walker, A.: The prediction of post-traumatic epilepsy. Archs Neurol. *36:* 8–12 (1979).

30 Cromptom, M.: Hypothalamic lesions following closed head injury. Brain *94:* 165–172 (1971).

31 Fleischer, A.; Rudman, D.; Payne, N.; Tindall, G.: Hypothalamic hypothyroidism and hypogonadism in prolonged traumacti coma. J. Neurosurg. *49:* 650–657 (1978).

32 Paxson, C.; Brown, D.: Post-traumatic anterior hypopituitarism. Pediatrics, Springfield *57:* 893–896 (1976).

33 Girard, J.; Marelli, R.: Posttraumatic hypothalamo-pituitary insufficiency. J. Pediat. *90:* 241–242 (1977).

34 Russell, W.; Nathan, P.: Traumatic amnesia. Brain *69:* 183–187 (1946).

35 Russell, W.: The traumatic amnesias (Oxford University Press, New York 1971).

36 Meyer, A.: The anatomical facts and clinical varieties of traumatic insanity. Am. J. Insan. *60:* 374–388 (1904).

37 Schilder, P.: Psychic disturbances after head injuries. Am. J. Psychiat. *91:* 155–188 (1934).

38 Adler, A.: Mental symptoms following head injury. A statistical analysis of two hundred cases. Archs Neurol. Psychiat. *53:* 34–43 (1945).

39 Teasdale, G.; Jennett, B.: Assessment of coma and impaired consciousness: a practical scale. Lancet *ii:* 81–84 (1974).

40 Levin, H.; O'Donnell, V.; Grossman, R.: The Galveston orientation and amnesia test: a practical scale to assess cognition after head injury. J. nerv. ment. dis. *167:* 675–684 (1979).

41 Overall, J.; Gorham, D.: The brief psychiatric rating scale. Psychol. Rep. *10:* 799–812 (1962).

42 Levin, H.; Grossman, R.: Behavioral sequelae of closed head injury. A quantitive study. Archs Neurol. *35:* 720–722 (1978).

43 Hall, R.; Popkin, M.; DeVaul, R.; Faillace, L.; Stickney, S.: Physical illness presenting as psychiatric disease. Archs gen. Psychiat. *35:* 1315–1320 (1978).

44 Hall, R.; Gruzenski, W.; Popkin, M.: Differential diagnosis of somatopsychic disorders. Psychosomatics *20:* 381–389 (1979).

45 Ommaya, A.; Gennarelli, T.: Cerebral concussion and traumatic unconsciousness:

correlation of experimental and clinical observations on blunt head injuries. Brain *97:* 633–654 (1974).

46 Brown, J.; Stoudemire, A.: Normal and pathological grief. J. Am. med. Ass. *250:* 378–382 (1983).

47 Weiner, M.; Caldwell, T: Stresses and coping in ICU nursing. II. Nurse support groups on intensive care units. Gen. Hosp. Psychiat. *3:* 129–134 (1981).

48 Diagnostic and statistical manual of mental disorders; 3rd ed., p. 104 (American Psychiatric Association, Washington 1980).

49 Lipowski, Z.: Delirium, clouding of consciousness and confusion. J. nerv. ment. Dis. *145:* 227–255 (1967).

50 Brown, C.: The alcohol withdrawal syndrome. Ann. Emerg. Med. *11:* 276–280 (1982).

51 Zisook, S.; DeVaul, R.: Adverse behavioral effects of benzodiazepines. J. fam. Prac. *5:* 963–966 (1977).

52 Khantzian, E.; McKenna, G.: Acute toxic and withdrawal reactions associated with drug use and abuse. Ann. intern. Med. *90:* 361–372 (1979).

53 Lishman, W.: Organic psychiatry. The psychological consequences of cerebral disorder (Blackwell, Oxford 1978).

54 Perl, M.; Peterson, L.; Dudrick, S.: Psychiatric problems encountered during intravenous nutrition; in Hill, Nutrition and the surgical patient, clinical surgery international, No. 2 (Churchill-Livingston, New York 1981).

55 Dudley, D.; Rowlett, D.; Loebel, P.: Emergency use of intravenous haloperidol. Gen. Hops. Psychiat. *1:* 240–246 (1979).

56 Feeney, D.; Gonzalez, A.; Law, W.: Amphetamine, haloperidol, and experience interact to affect rate of recovery after motor cortex injury. Science *217:* 855–857 (1982).

57 Ayd, F.: Parenteral (IM/IV) droperidol for acutely disturbed behavior in psychotic and non-psychotic individuals. Int. Drug Ther. Newslett. *15:* 1–4 (1980).

58 Lion, J.; Azcarate, C.; Koepke, H.: Paradoxical rage reactions during psychotropic medication. Dis. nerv. Syst. *36:* 557–558 (1975).

59 Osburne, N.: Biology of serotonergic transmission (Wiley, Chichester 1981).

60 Kellams, J.; Klapper, M.; Small, J.: Trazodone, a new antidepressant: efficacy and safety in endogenous depression. J. clin. Psychiat. *40:* 390–395 (1979).

61 Richelson, E.: Tricyclic antidepressants and neurotransmitter receptors. Psychiat. Ann. *9:* 186–195 (1979).

62 Diagnostic and statistical manual of mental disorders; 3rd ed., p. 236 (American Psychiatric Association, Washington 1980).

63 Marshall, J.: The treatment of night terrors associated with the posttraumatic syndrome. Am. J. Psychiat. *132:* 293–295 (1975).

64 Stuss, D.; Alexander, M.; Lieberman, A.; Levine, H.: An extraordinary form of confabulation. Neurology, Minneap. *28:* 1166–1172 (1978).

65 Blumer, D.; Benson, D.: Personality changes with frontal and temporal lobe lesions; in Benson, Blumer, Psychiatric aspects of neurologic disease, pp. 151–170 (Grune & Stratton, New York 1975).

66 Gazzaniga, M.; Volpe, B.: Split-brain studies: implications for psychiatry; in Arieti, American handbook of psychiatry; 2nd ed., No. 7, pp. 25–45 (Basic Books, New York 1981).

67 Peterson, L.; O'Shanick, G.: Endocrine diseases presenting with psychiatric symptoms. Post-grad. Med. *77:* 233–239 (1985).
68 Heilman, K.: Neglect and related disorders; in Heilman, Valenstein, Clinical neuropsychology (Oxford University Press, New York 1979).
69 Hall, J.; Speilman, G.; Gennarelli, T.: Auditory evoked responses in acute severe head injury. J. Neurosurg. Nurs. *14:* 225–231 (1982).
70 Diagnostic and statistical manual of mental disorders; 3rd ed., p. 118 (American Psychiatric Association, Washington 1980).
71 Diagnostic and statistical manual of mental disorders; 3rd ed., p. 295 (American Psychiatric Association, Washington 1980).
72 Ervin, E.; Mark, V.: Violence and the brain (Harper & Row, New York 1970).
73 Monroe, R.: Anticonvulsants in the treatment of aggression. J. nerv. ment. Dis. *160:* 119–126 (1975).
74 Tunks, E.; Dermer, S.: Carbamazepine in the dyscontrol syndrome associated with limbic system dysfunction. J. nerv. ment. Dis. *164:* 156 (1977).
75 Yudofsky, S.; Williams, D.; Gorman, J.: Propranolol in the treatment of rage and violent behavior in patients with chronic brain syndrome. Am. J. Psychiat. *138:* 218–220 (1981).
76 Cutler, N.; Heiser, J.: Retrospective diagnosis of hypomania following successful treatment of episodic violence with lithium. A case report. Am. J. Psychiat. *135:* 753–754 (1978).
77 Brown, G.; Ballanger, J.; Minichiello, M.; Goodwin, F.: Human aggression and its relationship to cerebrospinal fluid 5-hydroxyindoleacetic acid, 3-methoxy 4-hydroxyphenylglycol, and homovanillic acid; in Sadler, Psychopharmacology of aggression (Raven Press, New York 1979).
78 Richmond, J.; Young, J.; Groves, J.: Violent dyscontrol responsive to *d*-amphetamine. Am. J. Psachiat. *135:* 365–366 (1978).
79 Remick, R.; Fine, S.: Antipsychotic drugs and seizures. J. clin. Psychiat. *40:* 78–80 (1979).
80 Merskey, H.; Woodforde, J.: Psychiatric sequelae of minor head injury. Brain *95:* 521–528 (1972).
81 Diagnostic and statistical manual of mental disorders; 3rd ed., p. 117 (American Psychiatric Association, Washington 1980).
82 Lishman, W.: The psychiatric sequelae of head injury. A review. Psychol. Med. *3:* 304–318 (1973).
83 Asberg, M.: Plasma nortriptyline levels – relationship to clinical effects. Clin. Pharmacol. Ther. *16:* 215–229 (1974).
84 Amsterdam, J.; Brunswick, D.; Mendels, J.: The clinical application of tricyclic antidepressant pharmacokinetics and plasma levels. Am. J. Psychiat. *137:* 653–662 (1980).
85 Lipsey, J.; Robinson, R.; Pearlson, G.; Rao, K.; Price, T.: Nortriptyline treatment of post-stroke depression. A double-blind study. Lancet *i:* 297–300 (1984).
86 Gershon, S.; Newton, R.: Lack of anticholinergic side effects with a new antidepressant – trazodone. J. clin. Psychiat. *41:* 100–104 (1980).
87 Goldberg, E.; Gerstman, L.; Mattis, S.; Hughes, J.; Bilder, R.; Sirio, C.: Effects of cholinergic treatment on posttraumatic anterograde amnesia. Archs Neurol. *39:* 581 (1982).

88   Brooks, D.; McKinlay, W.: Personality and behavioural change after severe blunt head injury – a relative's view. J. Neurol. Neurosurg. Psychiat. *46:* 336–344 (1983).

89   Rosenbaum, M.; Najenson, J.: Changes in life pattern and symptoms of low mood as reported by wives of severely brain injuried soldiers. J. consult. clin. Pychol. *44:* 881–888 (1976).

90   Thomsen, I: Late outcome of very severe blunt head trauma. A 10–15 year second follow-up. J. Neurol. Neurosurg. Psychiat. *47:* 260–268 (1984).

91   Holland, L.: Whalley, M.: The work of the psychiatrist in a rehabilitation hospital. Br. J. Psychiat. *138:* 222–229 (1981).

92   Groves, J.: Taking care of the hateful patient. New Engl. J. Med. *298:* 883–887 (1978).

Gregory J. O'Shanick, MD, Medical Psychiatry Service, Medical College of Virginia, Richmond, VA 23298 (USA)

Adv. psychosom. Med., vol. 16, pp. 194–229 (Karger, Basel 1986)

Rehabilitation of Cognitive and Behavioral Dysfunction in Head Injury

Mary Ellen Hayden, Tessa Hart

Medical Center Del Oro, Houston, Tex., USA

Until recently, rehabilitation of head injury meant remediating as many of the physical problems as possible and then discharging the patient. Statistics clearly show that the outcome after such treatment is bleak. The probability of successful return to competitive employment after a severe head injury is low, with long-term disability being the result of residual physical disability in a minority of cases [1]. The remainder of the disabled head injured victims are unable to work because of cognitive and behavioral problems. Personality changes and diminished ability to sustain satisfactory adult relationships result in a significant degree of burden on the family [2].

In this chapter we will review the most common neuroanatomical, cognitive, and behavioral defects after head injury, and describe state-of-the-art procedures for the rehabilitation of cognitive, behavioral, and emotional coping dysfunctions in the various stages of recovery. We will conclude with some comments on the importance of an interdisciplinary team approach to the rehabilitation of the head-injured adult.

Typical Neuropsychological Residua of Head Injury

A comprehensive discussion of the pathophysiological effects of closed head injury is provided in the chapter by *O'Shanick* [this issue]. Even more detailed reviews of this subject are presented by *Jennett and Teasdale* [3] and by *Levin* et al. [4].

Motor, cognitive, and behavioral deficits following closed head injury would naturally reflect those neuroanatomical structures which have been affected by the injury. Motor dysfunction would be common because of the high frequency of diffuse white matter tearing in the pons, cerebellum, and internal capsule. Cognitive and behavioral deficits would be secondary to: (1) diffuse white matter shearing at different levels of the neuraxis; (2) hemispheric disconnection syndromes (due to callosal shearing); (3) any focal lesions, including frontotemporal contusions and intracerebral hematomae, and (4) any diffuse gray matter damage (in cases with secondary ischemic hypoxia, increased intracranial pressure, and/or diffuse edema).

In organizing a detailed discussion of cognitive and behavioral deficits, the neuropsychological framework developed by *Luria* [5] is frequently helpful. *Luria* emphasized the importance of avoiding a strict localizationist orientation to correlating specific mental activities with specific neuroanatomical substrates. He adopted instead a systems approach, focusing on interactions among various structures in carrying out a cognitive/behavioral function. *Luria's* orientation is particularly useful in discussing cognitive/behavioral changes after closed head injury because: (1) the differential distribution of contusions appears maximally to affect some neuropsychological *systems* as compared with others, and (2) the diffuse shearing of the white matter tends to disrupt the connections between various structures, disturbing many *systems* of cognitive/behavioral functions.

Luria conceptualizes human neuropsychological functioning as being divisible into three principal systems or 'functional units'. Functional unit I is primarily responsible for regulating arousal, alertness, and 'cortical tone'. Neuroanatomically, it is primarily subcortical and includes the so-called 'nonspecific' systems in the brain stem and thalamus, the limbic system, and the orbital and mesial frontal lobes. Functional unit II is primarily responsible for obtaining, processing, and storing information. It is subserved by specific sensory nuclei of the thalamus and the posterior convexity of the cerebral hemispheres, including those areas which process visual, auditory, and other sensory information. Functional unit III is primarily responsible for programming, regulating, and verifying both overt and covert behavior. Its chief neuroanatomical substrate is the convexity of the frontal areas of the cerebral hemispheres.

Units I and III would appear to be relatively more vulnerable to the direct effects of closed head injury because of the high incidence

of contusions in the temporal and frontal areas. Unit II appears
less vulnerable, although shearing effects would be expected to result
in: (1) an overall information processing limitation which would affect
all unit II modalities, and (2) possible disconnections among the
various structures. The following discussion presents the literature
on cognitive and behavioral deficits after head injury in the context
of *Luria's* three functional units. For the purpose of economy our
review is selective rather than exhaustive, and certain points have been
simplified.

Functional Unit I:
The Unit for Regulating Cortical Tone

In discussing this unit, *Luria* [5] quotes *Pavlov's* statement: 'Organized, goal-directed activity requires maintenance of an optimal level
of cortical tone' (p. 44). All cognitive functioning is highly dependent
upon the precise regulation of cortical tone by these systems, and
disruption in the functioning of this unit results in many of the profound cognitive and behavioral dysfunctions typically seen after closed
head injury. In particular, coma, post-traumatic amnesia, attentional
deficits, and memory dysfunction are among the most common neuropsychological sequelae of head injury.

Coma
Coma of immediate onset is typically the result of shearing effects
which reach the level of the mesencephalic brainstem and disrupt the
reticular activating system [6, 7]. *Ommaya and Gennarelli* [6] found that
loss of consciousness was typically associated with significant rotational forces, whereas purely linear forces did not induce coma. Because of
the centripetal sequence of shear strain, disruption of mesencephalic
structures is believed to be present only with widespread injury to the
cerebral hemispheres [8, 9]. An exception to this rule is found in cases
where traumatic hyperextension of the head causes contusions and
hemorrhage at the pontomedullary junction extending rostrally into the
pons but without involvement of the cerebral hemispheres [10]. In
general, however, different coma durations are believed to reflect varying degrees of diffuse axonal injury such that a lengthy coma suggests
widespread, severe axonal damage [11].

Attention

Deficits in the ability to sustain attention have been ascribed to head injured patients since the work of *Conkey* [12]. *Luria* describes functional unit I in terms of its task of modulating and regulating the tonic states of the cerebral cortex to allow evaluation of incoming stimuli to determine whether or not they are novel and, further, whether they require attention. The neuropsychological literature implicates the reticular systems of the brain as the principal structures underlying this function, although integrity of the entire brain is probably necessary for maximal efficiency. *Van Zomeren* et al. [13] provide an excellent review of the literature on the attentional sequelae of closed head injury. Their own work, based on a cognitive or information-processing approach to attention, suggests that:

(1) Tonic alertness, or the ability to sustain vigilance over time, does not appear to be diminished in head injured individuals. In fact, there is some suggestion that *a supranormal tonic level* of alertness is typical of closed head injury patients. This may represent a compensatory coping mechanism which seeks constantly to overcome cognitive deficits.

(2) *Phasic alertness,* or more rapid changes dependent on interests and intentions, appears to be impaired after closed head injury. This suggests that a patient's preparedness for appropriate action is suboptimal.

(3) Distraction has a disproportionate effect on head-injured patients. However, no compelling evidence supports the idea of a deficit of focused attention. As an alternative hypothesis, patients may be *slower in dealing with interference from irrelevant stimuli.*

(4) If attention is defined in terms of speed of processing (i.e. the amount of data processed over a unit of time), patients are clearly at a disadvantage when compared with normal controls. Slow processing appears to be primarily due to a *decreased rate of central processing,* although there is also evidence for slowed perceptual and motor functioning.

Tying these cognitive functions directly to neuroanatomical lesions after head injury is, of course, not possible. However, *Van Zomeren* et al. [13] provide an interesting discussion of the various structures which have been implicated in slowed processing in brain-damaged individuals. *Gronwall and Sampson* [14] suggested that brain stem lesions are responsible for these findings. However, as was previously discussed, brain stem lesions are rare without concomitant shearing in the cerebral hemispheres, making tenuous any attribution of these deficits to the brain stem alone. In addition, slowed processing and attentional deficits occur with mild head injuries [15] where brain stem lesions are even less likely. Biochemical alterations have been invoked to explain the attentional disturbances [16] as have lesions in the basal ganglia and cerebral cortex [13]. Following a Lurian approach and adding evidence from *Ommaya* [17], a disruption in connections between the cortical frontotemporal zones and the diencephalic reticular systems could contribute to disruption in attentional processes. Insufficient data exist for determining which, if any, of these hypotheses is correct.

Memory

Another major system within *Luria's* functional unit I is that subserving memory functioning. The neuroanatomical structures believed to be critical for the acquisition of new memories lie in the thalamus (i.e. dorsomedial nucleus) and the limbic system (i.e. hippocampus, fornix and mammillary bodies). Lesions restricted to these areas are known to produce three common deficits: (1) anterograde amnesia; (2) varying degrees of retrograde amnesia, and (3) confabulation, all in the context of relatively preserved intellectual functioning [18]. A shrinking retrograde amnesia and impaired memory for ongoing daily events (with or without confabulation) are common sequelae of closed head injury and are given the name 'post-traumatic amnesia'. The length of post-traumatic amnesia is believed to be positively correlated with the extent of brain damage [11] and negatively correlated with eventual outcome (however, see *Brooks* [19] for a discussion of the methodological flaws complicating the interpretation of this literature).

Most of the literature on memory dysfunction after head injury addresses the period after recovery from post-traumatic amnesia. Reviews of this literature by *Levin* et al. [4] and *Brooks* [19] suggest significant residual deficits long after the resolution of post-traumatic amnesia and, in fact, after the recovery of many other cognitive functions to approximately premorbid levels. *Levin* et al. conclude that short-term auditory memory may be disrupted in patients who remain disoriented, but is otherwise fairly resistant to the effects of head injury. In contrast, long-term memory for new information is more vulnerable. *Levin* et al. also suggest that old, prelearned information is relatively invulnerable to head injury, but storage and retrieval of new information becomes particularly problematic. *Brook's* [19] summary is similar, suggesting that studies which use very simple measures of immediate memory (e.g. digits forward) report marked recovery within 3 years or less, often up to a normal level. However, studies of verbal learning generally show slow recovery and marked deficits up to at least a year.

In our own clinical experience, based on following several hundred head-injured patients over several years, 'memory problems' are among the most frequent and persistent complaints of patients, families, teachers, and employers. These complaints frequently appear disproportionate to the problems we would anticipate based on the results of neuropsychological testing, even using such sensitive instruments as the Buschke Selective Reminding procedure [20] and the Continuous Recognition Memory Test [21]. We have been surprised by many patients who perform within normal limits on formal memory testing but who exhibit a significant degree of dysfunction typically attributed to 'poor memory' while at work or elsewhere outside of the clinic setting. Whether this reflects a true failure of 'memory' is difficult to determine. As a matter of fact, we have long suspected an information capacity limit as the basis of these problems. This is consistent with the thoughts of *Van Zomeren* et al. [13], who point out the relationship between speed of processing and the formation of memory traces: If information is processed at a slower than average rate, the amount of information which gets processed and stored over any unit of time will be less. *Brooks* [19] also suspects a quantitative rather than qualitative difference between the memory functioning of head-injured patients and controls. This framework certainly accomodates our observation that many patients can perform well in familiar, highly structured environments but become 'overloaded' in settings which require more rapid processing of novel information.

Personality

Luria's functional unit I also plays an important role in emotionality. *Schacter* [22] postulates that the experience of emotion is dependent upon an interaction between arousal and an appropriate cognitive state. In their discussion of mental sequelae after head injury, *Jennett and Teasdale* [3] note that cognitive deficits are almost always accompanied by patient and/or family perceptions of 'personality changes'. However, the perception of personality changes does not always have an identifiable basis in cognitive change. Some of these affective sequelae may well be the result of deficits in the arousal component of emotionality. *Valenstein and Heilman* [23] point out that this component depends heavily upon structures in the corticolimbic-reticular loop. In particular, the cingulate, hippocampus, fornix, mammillary bodies, anterior and dorsomedial thalamus, hypothalamus, orbito-frontal, insular and anterior temporal cortical regions, and amygdala have been included in this system. Animal experimentation has shown that stimulation of the amygdala produces rage reactions or gross increases in emotionality, whereas ablation of that structure results in a placid animal. The opposite is true of the septal area where lesions produce rage reactions and stimulation produces a pleasant state that animals will work to induce. Based on human studies, *Damasio and Van Hoesen* [24] note that massive lesions in the anterior cingulate area often produce akinetic mutism, which can be interpreted as a severe inability to appreciate or express emotions. Partial lesions result in decreased anxiety and agitation. The hypothalamus also appears to have an important role in the arousal component of emotionality and appetitive behavior [25]. *Damasio and Van Hoesen* [24] suggest that emotional disturbances after limbic lesions do not appear in isolation, but are typically associated with defects in general activity level, diminished memory functioning, or impaired social behavior. Considering the high probability of limbic system disruption in head injured individuals, 'personality changes' in the form of increases or decreases in overall emotional tone should be common.

Functional Unit II: The Unit for Receiving, Analyzing, and Storing Information

Luria's second functional unit is subserved primarily by the posterior convexity of the cerebral hemispheres and includes the visual, auditory, and other sensory systems. Each of these systems is arranged in a hierarchical structure with primary and secondary components. The primary or projection area of each system is highly modality specific (responsive only to input from a particular sensory modality) and displays a one-to-one topological correspondence between points in the sensory field and points in the neural substrate. For example, a discrete lesion in the primary visual cortex results in a discrete loss of vision in the corresponding portion of the visual field. Direct interhemispheric connections are minimal between the primary areas, and no lateral specialization exists at this level. Secondary areas are also highly specific with regard to particular sensory modalities, but more analysis and elaboration of sensory information occurs at this level. For example, a lesion in the secondary visual cortical region would result in a visual perceptual deficit rather than a field defect. Interhemispheric communication is more plentiful, and lateral specialization is evident at this level. The tertiary areas of unit II integrate input from the various sensory systems and as such are not modality specific. Interhemispheric connections are rich, and lateral specialization is complex. Considering the typical diffuse white matter lesions post head injury in the context of *Luria's* second functional unit, one would expect a general loss of efficiency in any or all of the systems within this unit due to: (1) diminution of input to the unit from lower brain structures; (2) less efficient communication among the various structures within the unit, and (3) diminished interhemispheric communication because of callosal lesions. In addition, disturbances within the first functional unit would undoubtedly result in less efficient maintenance of the ongoing cortical tone necessary for efficient processing within unit II. Secondary gray matter destruction as the result of hypoxia, etc., would further affect the efficiency of these systems. Focal lesions, if present, would result in specific neuropsychological deficits associated with the specific site of the lesion. However, macroscopic lesions of the convex surface, particularly in the occipital portion of this unit, are rare in the absence of a depressed skull fracture [26]. Research to date has shown the following unit II sequelae of head injury.

Visual

Specific primary visual deficits occurring after head injury appear most frequently to be the result of injury to the optic nerve rather than higher in the primary visual system [27, 28]. *Ruesch* [29] presents some research which appears to reflect the effect of diffuse white matter damage on visual processing speed for information presented tachistoscopically. He found that the minimum exposure time necessary for perception of three-digit numbers was increased by 142% in recently head-injured individuals and by 33% in patients with chronic injuries. *Hannay* et al. [30] obtained further evidence of processing delays for discrete visual information using a similar paradigm. *Levin* et al. [4] point out the paucity of other studies of perceptual deficits after head injury, citing only one other study in which a head-injured patient demonstrated prosopagnosia (an inability to recognize familiar faces) for several months post-injury. This patient initially exhibited visuospatial impairments, memory defects, and hypersexuality, but by 1 year post-injury the prosopagnosia had recovered (although the visuospatial deficits remained).

Auditory

Hearing loss due to auditory nerve damage is relatively frequent after head injury (8% of cases) [27]. Information is lacking on other auditory deficits after head injury.

Somatosensory

An analysis of complex tactile abilities was performed by *Dikmen* et al. [32] with the finding of significant diminution of performance on the Tactual Performance Test as long as 18 months post-injury.

Language

Discrimination of basic speech sounds (phonemes), language comprehension, and reading are important functions subserved by the posterior tertiary area, particularly in the left hemisphere. Classical posterior aphasic syndromes (such as Wernicke's aphasia) are rare in the absence of focal lesions. A relatively small proportion of patients demonstrate other linguistic dysfunctions such as word finding difficulties and impaired comprehension of complex commands [4]. With regard to reading, it is our clinical experience that severely injured head trauma patients seldom 'read for fun', perhaps because of subtle residual attentional deficits, but that dyslexia per se is extremely rare.

Personality

There are some special functions within unit II associated with the posterior cortical regions, particularly of the right hemisphere, which if disturbed could be manifested as a 'personality change'. The perception of emotion based on intonational patterns of speech appears to be particularly disrupted in individuals who have sustained right temporoparietal infarctions, as compared to those with similar left hemispheric lesions who exhibit a receptive aphasia [33]. Similarly, *Valenstein and Heilman* [23] suggest that the visual perceptual problems which frequently occur with right posterior cerebral damage result in impairments in the ability to interpret facial affect. Clearly, either of these cognitive changes could be misunderstood as a decrease in sensitivity to the feelings of family and friends.

Functional Unit III: The Unit for Programming, Regulating, and Verifying

Luria's third functional unit primarily involves the structures in the anterior regions of the cerebral hemispheres. This unit has a hierarchical organization analogous to that of the second functional unit. The primary motor cortex is the point of origin of the pyramidal tract which is mapped one-on-one to parts of the body. The secondary motor area 'prepares the motor programmes' to be initiated by the primary motor cortex. The tertiary portion of this unit, the prefrontal divisions of the brain, plays a crucial role in the formation of intentions and plans and in the regulation and verification of the most complex forms of behavior. The tertiary area has very rich connections with other cortical structures, with the subcortical limbic system, and with the basal ganglia [34, 35]. It plays important roles in activation and inhibition at the highest level through its connections with the reticular systems, and in regulatory functions such as initiation, maintenance, and termination of movement through the two lower divisions of the motor cortex.

In terms of higher cognitive function, the tertiary portions of unit III exert modulatory controls allowing for the planning, execution, and evaluation of complex responses. *Damasio* [34] points out that this portion of the frontal lobes allows for maximal structural separation between stimulus (S) and response (R), allowing the nervous system to go beyond reflex activity. He states, 'What lies between S and R is a complex chain of decisions, such as how to process S to the best advantage and how to respond to S in the way more suitable to the set of immediate and long-term goals of the individual' (p. 369). He further states that 'it is the ability to handle hypercomplex environmental contingencies in the framework of the individual's own history, and in the perspective of his desired future course, that distinguishes frontal-lobe operation' (p. 370). Since the tertiary areas of unit III modulate more primitive forms of response, lesions in these regions would be expected to result in a diminution of response elaboration. Hypokinesis and initiation problems, perseveration, and decrements in the performance of sequential coordinated movements are, in fact, very common in the acute phases following head injury.

In summarizing the neuropsychological deficits which occur as a result of frontal lobe damage, *Lezak* [36] states that the characteristic intellectual impairment does not involve a loss of specific skills, information, or problem-solving abilities. Rather, frontal lobe dysfunction is more clearly manifested in unstructured situations. With regard to intellectual abilities after head injury, *Mandleberg and Brooks* [37] found a greater decrement in performance IQ than in verbal IQ as measured by the WAIS, and a slower recovery of these nonverbal functions. The verbal IQ had improved to within the average range at approximately 1 year post-injury in their series, while performance IQ continued to recover over a 3-year period. These findings may be attributed to the greater complexity of performance than of verbal items, the latter of which typically require overlearned, readily elicited responses. Performance items, on the other hand, involve novel stimuli and require the integration of a number of functions including perception, learning, manual dexterity, speed, and extended periods of attention. *Dikmen* et al. [32] demonstrated diminished performance on trails A and B and on the Halstead Category Test 18 months post-injury. These tests involve a high degree of planning, hypothesis generation and testing, and response shifting.

Personality
Damage to the prefrontal cortical regions has long been associated with a variety of characteristic personality changes [35]. In cases of mild impairment traceable to frontal lobe involvement, personality change may in fact be the only detectable consequence of the injury. *Lezak* [36] lists five major behavioral disturbances secondary to frontal lobe damage, each easily characterized as an alteration in personality. Difficulties in *initiation* often appear as decreased spontaneity, decreased productivity, or loss of motivation and 'drive'. Deficits in the *shifting of responses* (whether at the motoric, ideational, or attitudinal level) are frequently seen as rigidity. Difficulty in *stopping ongoing behavior* often results in impulsivity, disinhibition, or overreactivity. *Defective self-awareness* is frequently accompanied by euphoria, loss of normal anxiety, and lack of concern for social conventions. Finally, a *concrete*

attitude often precludes advance planning or foresight. 'Frontal lobe syndromes', as they involve loss of the basic monitoring and regulatory functions necessary for adaptive behavior in complex situations, are among the most dramatic examples of personality change following injury to the brain [38].

Summary. The most pronounced cognitive deficits after head injury appear to be those associated with *Luria's* functional unit I: Maintenance of ongoing cortical tone to support consistent and efficient attention; the ability consistently to lay down new memories; and the ability to maintain maximum functioning with distractions, under stress or fatigue, and with increasingly complex information processing demands. Clinicians experienced with this patient population are well aware that even years post-injury with relatively good recovery, patients continue to have difficulty functioning when fatigued or when they are in stressful, informationally complex situations. They experience considerable failure as a result of variability of performance across modalities, tasks, and settings. These cognitive deficits are frequently seen as 'personality changes' which alienate family and friends. Successful rehabilitation efforts must therefore address specific cognitive deficits in increasingly complex and stressful conditions. The manifestations of these cognitive deficits in interpersonal relationships is an equally important rehabilitation target. These issues are addressed in more detail below.

Cognitive and Behavioral Rehabilitation

Our discussion in this section will follow roughly the typical stages of recovery after severe injury, from coma to social and vocational reintegration. For each stage we will describe some of the interventions appropriate for the cognitive and behavioral sequelae of head trauma.

Coma

It may at first seem paradoxical to consider the possibility of cognitive or behavioral remediation for the comatose patient. However, coma is not an all-or-none phenomenon but a continuum of neurological disruption which follows a more or less orderly progression of stages in the recovery of voluntary function [39]. It is tempting to think of these recovery stages as capable of 'acceleration', perhaps by direct modification of the neurological responsiveness of comatose patients.

One widespread idea, which has received a good deal of popular press as well as interest from rehabilitation specialists, is that certain types of 'stimulation' might accelerate recovery from coma. At some facilities for head injury rehabilitation, comatose patients are treated with 'sensory bombardment' programs involving the delivery of intense stimulation to one or more modalities [40]. This procedure seems to be based on the idea that the brain whose function is temporarily depressed will be 'forced' to accept environmental stimuli if they are of sufficient intensity. While this is an intuitively appealing notion, we know of no empirical data to support it. In fact, *Luria* et al. [41] caution against the use of 'strong and excessively strong' stimulation in the acute phases of recovery from head trauma. These investigators discuss the possibility that intense stimuli may actually not evoke a physiological response in the inhibited CNS, whereas moderate levels of stimulation would be expected to produce a normal response. Again, we know of no research evidence to support or refute either view. However, given this measure of doubt and in the absence of empirical data, the medical community would do well to treat sensory bombardment programs with a healthy skepticism.

We are aware of only two published reports describing specific attempts to modify the responsiveness of comatose patients. *Weber* [42] explored the effects of sensory stimulation (ice application, muscle stretching and tapping) on EEG in 3 patients who had been comatose for less than a week. Although her results were variable, there was some indication that normalization of EEG rhythms and sleep cycles and a clinically quieter appearance followed the stimulation sessions.

Boyle and Greer [43] worked with 3 patients who had been unresponsive for at least 6 months after the onset of coma. These investigators used an operant approach, attempting to increase the frequency of behaviors which were sometimes observed to follow verbal requests. Brief selections of the patients' favorite music were made contingent on performing certain movements of the eyes, mouth, or fingers on command. After several weeks of this training, the rate of the target behaviors appeared to increase in only 1 patient, and even in this case there was a great deal of variability from day to day. Interestingly, the 1 patient who did seem to respond to the procedure was the only 1 of the 3 who eventually recovered from coma; another remained in a persistent vegetative state, and the third died.

Until these types of remediations are studied more extensively, and until the effects of intense stimulation programs are understood, direct intervention for the comatose patient falls mostly under the rubric of medical management. The cognitive/behavioral specialist on a rehabilitation unit may assist in an indirect way by helping to monitor the responsivity of the patient and/or by providing necessary education, support, and counseling for the patient's family and caretakers. For example, the family of a comatose patient would benefit from understanding the nature and progression of stages in coma. Knowing that the time spent in a particular stage of recovery is of limited prognostic value [39] might reassure a relative who is anxiously comparing notes with the families of other patients. It is also important to be sensitive to difficulties experienced by nurses and other personnel responsible for the basic daily care of comatose patients. These workers may be prone to feelings of hopelessness, discouragement, and repulsion [44], all of which may easily be communicated unintentionally to the patient and family.

Agitation and Confusion

Patients who sustain a significant head injury, with or without coma, sometimes experience a stage of recovery marked by thrashing, combativeness, yelling, and excessive movement. This agitated state may persist for weeks, and may reappear later under conditions of extreme stress [45]. It has been our experience that the agitation following a prolonged coma presents a different clinical picture from that of patients who 'hit the ground and come up yelling'. The latter group, who become combative after a brief coma or no coma, tend to show more hyperactivity and to remain agitated for a longer period of time. We have not seen data on the anatomical or physiological correlates of the various clinical forms of agitation, but it may be speculated that these syndromes reflect different levels of CNS involvement. Possibly there is a greater degree of limbic system disruption in the case of a patient who is persistently belligerent and hyperactive without coma.

The agitated patient is a behavior management challenge partly because the behavior is dramatic, frightening, and easily misunderstood by both lay persons (e.g. family members) and rehabilitation specialists.

Cognitive/behavioral intervention at this stage consists of efforts to structure the patients' environment to minimize the degree and frequency of agitated responses and, once again, education and counseling for the patient's family and caretakers. The most effective behavioral management strategy for agitation may be summarized as follows: Offering a calm, safe, reassuring environment works better than isolation or restraint, which may actually exacerbate the problem [46, 47]. *Olson and Henig* [48] and *Malkmus* [47] offer some useful general suggestions for dealing with the agitated patient: (1) notice what triggers the agitated response, and eliminate it from the environment; (2) notice what calms the patient, and provide it; (3) allow patients to walk and talk, and (4) redirect the patient's attention away from the source of the agitation. It is probably useless to expect an agitated patient to participate in a formal schedule of therapy, although he or she should be given an opportunity to engage in a variety of activities (particularly gross motor activities), switching frequently from one to the next. It should always be remembered that agitation takes different clinical forms and that a soothing stimulus for one patient may aggravate another. For example, we have noticed that despite the cautions against isolation, some patients are calmer when they are alone in a quiet room and become most agitated when approached by another person.

The pharmacological management of this phase of recovery is a somewhat controversial issue. In order to control restless and combative behavior, psychotropic medication must often be given in doses so large as to produce sedation, with a general suppression of cognitive function. There is also some experimental evidence to suggest that haloperidol, which is frequently prescribed for post-traumatic agitation, may slow the natural recovery process under some circumstances [49]. In general, management of this type of agitation with pharmacologic agents should be considered only after the failure of carefully planned behavioral and environmental interventions.

The treatment of agitation may be enhanced in an indirect way through the counseling of the patient's family, who are in critical need of education regarding a recovery phase which to the lay person resembles 'crazy behavior' or 'misbehavior'. The family needs to know that the agitation is temporary and that it represents a step towards recovery [47]. Their cooperation can greatly enhance the effectiveness of management at this stage, since the presence of familiar and well-liked people helps to alleviate agitation [48]. Nurses and other medical personnel caring for patients in this stage also need to understand the nature of agitation. *Fauman* [46] presents a scenario in which belligerence, uncooperativeness, 'and other unacceptable personality changes often appear to the medical staff to be under the conscious control of the patient' (p. 381), particularly when the disturbance is intermittent. Staff members may respond with anger at the patient, guilt at their own anger, and avoidance of the source of guilt (the patient), all of which would exacerbate the agitation by isolating the patient.

Whether they become agitated or not, patients recovering from a head injury severe enough to induce coma may be expected to exhibit confusional states of varying duration. During the period of post-traumatic amnesia, patients are disoriented to time and place, fail to remember ongoing events, and show a variety of cognitive and behavioral disturbances [50]. During this phase, as with agitation, the most fruitful approaches to direct remediation are those which concentrate on structuring the patient's environment in order to minimize the impact of the confusion. As far as possible, the number of different environments (e.g. therapy settings) used by the patients should be limited, as should the presence of distraction within an environment [47]. The therapeutic milieu should be routinized and consistent, with as few surprises as possible. Repetition to the point of dullness, particularly considering the learning deficits of the amnesic patient, will be more effective than bombardment with a variety of activities [48]. Rehabilitation team members must also be counseled not to expect carryover of learning from one setting to another; parallel training in all settings is an important team goal at this stage.

The treatment of confused/amnesic patients can be extremely difficult for several reasons. First, almost by definition these patients are unaware of the circumstances of their injuries, and they may deny the need for (or actually resist) hospitalization and treatment. Second, partly as a byproduct of the pathophysiology of head trauma, behavioral disinhibition and various forms of 'social inappropriateness' are extremely common in the acute stages of recovery following coma. In a provocative article entitled *Hate in the Rehabilitation Setting, Gans* [51] discusses the 'devastating' effect on even experienced staff members of working day after day with patients 'devoid of the civilizing contributions of the frontal and temporal lobes' (p. 178). Among the patient responses contributing to staff burnout, *Gans* cites denial of disability, lack of recognition for team members' efforts (partly secondary to amnesia), and sexual disinhibition as being particularly insidious. He recommends institutionalized structures to improve staff morale on acute rehabilitation units, and team education on the reasons for patient's behaviors and appropriate ways to set limits.

Post-Acute Cognitive and Behavioral Sequelae

As we have discussed earlier, closed head injury brings with it a constellation of cognitive and behavioral changes which are, on the one hand, highly characteristic of the disorder and on the other hand, variable depending on such factors as severity of the injury, focal brain lesions, and premorbid experience. After the acute stages of recovery from head injury (coma, agitation and/or confusion, and post-traumatic amnesia), the emphasis of rehabilitation shifts from that of ensuring medical stability and a structured environment to more active remediations for cognitive and behavioral deficits. We recognize that in a clinical sense, post-traumatic changes in cognition, behavior, and personality can never be fully disentangled from one another or from the effects of the individual's attempts to cope with perceived changes. For the purposes of discussion, however, we will review the various therapeutic modalities that have been developed for cognitive dysfunctions separately from issues more relevant to understanding changes in personality and behavior.

Remediations for Cognitive Dysfunction

It has been only recently that neuropsychologists and other behavioral specialists have begun to attempt the 'direct' remediation of deficits in attention, memory, and other higher cognitive functions in brain-injured patients. Most of these remediations (collectively referred to as 'cognitive retraining') involve providing practice on structured tasks which exercise the defective skill or promote the acquisition of new cognitive strategies. Training procedures to compensate for defective memory were among the first to be developed and continue to attract a good deal of experimentation. For example, patients with left hemisphere damage have been taught to use visual imagery to compensate for verbal memory deficits [52–56]. Other investigators have trained brain-injured patients to use the construction of sentences or stories to assist in the recall of word lists [56–60]. While most of these studies report some success (i.e. enhanced recall) after training, very few have followed subjects for more than a few days and even fewer report controlled data on the effect of training on subjects' everyday memory functioning.

Various aspects of language function have also been the focus of this type of intervention. *Luria* and his colleagues [41, 61] present a detailed discussion of the retraining of complex skills such as reading, writing, articulation, and comprehension based on a functional analysis of the intact and defective links in the skill system. *Albert* et al. [62] report the use of a speech therapy technique known as melodic intonation therapy, which capitalizes on relatively intact singing ability to enhance speech production in severely dysfluent aphasics. In an ingenious study, *Gardner* et al. [63] taught a rudimentary nonverbal 'language' using tokens of different shapes and colors to global aphasics who had failed to improve with conventional speech therapy.

The retraining of visual perceptual skills has been extensively studied in patients with left hemispatial neglect as a consequence of right hemisphere damage. Both improvement with practice on specially designed scanning exercises and generalization of training to other activities have been reported [64, 65]. The effects of practice on visual analysis and discrimination tasks, however, may be more subtle with regard to clinically significant improvement [66].

In considering the issue of direct cognitive retraining for the patient with closed head injury, several aspects of this literature should be borne in mind. First, few of these retraining methods have been formally tested with head-injured subjects. Nearly all of the controlled studies reporting success have been carried out with stroke patients who, presumably, have at least one well-functioning cerebral hemisphere. In fact, some of the reports cited above include caveats regarding the failure of their methods in subjects with bilateral, mesial, or extensive frontal involvement [52, 57]. Recalling our earlier discussion, it would appear that most cognitive remediations have been developed and tested for patients with primary dysfunction in *Luria's* second functional unit, the brain systems responsible for handling sensory information. The head-injured patient, as we have seen, is primarily vulnerable to disruption in medial systems handling attention and speed of processing (*Luria's* unit I) and overall behavioral regulation (unit III). Focal deficits associated with lateralized damage are either absent or 'superimposed' on the typical clinical picture of information processing inefficiency. Therefore, it would be naive to expect a technique successful for stroke patients to be equally effective for the closed head injury population. Our experience has been, instead, that these specific retraining techniques benefit head-injured patients only with extensive modification.

The second aspect of the cognitive retraining literature which must be considered is the content of the remedial activities which have so far been developed. Many of these techniques have been based on a psychometric model, such that patients are essentially taught strategies for improving their scores on tests of list learning [53] or constructional praxis [67]. The assumption is that such training will transfer to activities more meaningful to the patient's everyday life. However, the relationships between specific patterns of test performance and other domains of behavior are still far from clear [68, 69]. Even demonstrations of the correlations among defective test performances and impairments in activities of daily living do not necessarily imply that treating one will have any effect on the other.

Our own approach to cognitive retraining with closed-head-injured patients assumes that the *content* of training should include skills that the patient needs for future success at home, on the job, or in the community. The *process* by which these skills are taught reflects our assumption that the basic cognitive deficit in cases of severe closed head injury is one of information processing. Thus, each skill taught in our cognitive remediation programs is analyzed with regard to its information processing demands; these are, in turn, systematically increased over time so that eventually the skill is performed under approximately naturalistic conditions. For example, a basic skill such as food preparation might be taught using exercises in the following sequence: (1) answering questions based on a simple package label; (2) answering questions from memory, based on finding the information on the appropriate part of an actual food package; (3) preparing the contents of a food package according to the directions, and (4) coordinating the sequence of several recipes to prepare a full meal. The patient would be required to master the tasks at each level before attempting activities under conditions of *less* structure and cueing and *more* complexity and stress.

Treatment of Personality and Behavioral Dysfunction

As we have seen, the acute phases of recovery from severe head injury are frequently marked by florid changes in affect and behavior such as agitation and restlessness or hypoactivity with extreme apathy and flatness [50]. Following the resolution of the acute confusional state, it is still extremely common to find persistent alterations in affect or behavior which are interpreted as 'personality changes' by the patient or his family and friends. By the first year or two following the injury, significant personality changes are reported by at least two-thirds of severely head-injured patients or their families [70, 71]. The most frequently mentioned sequelae include irritability and difficulties with impulse control, dependency, loss of energy and initiative, and various manifestations of egocentricity [25, 71]. Anxiety and depression are also common [72]. These and other changes serve to exacerbate the social isolation and withdrawal reported by these patients [72, 73].

In order to attempt intervention for these common and extremely handicapping difficulties, it is important to understand the complex nature of their origins. Changes in personality or behavior after a severe head injury are determined by a network of interactive factors including: The direct effects of the brain injury; the patient's attempts to compensate for, and cope with, changes in cognitive, physical, and emotional status; and factors in the environment which help to shape affective and behavioral responses. All of these factors interact with aspects of the premorbid personality to produce the clinical picture seen at any given time post-trauma.

In the first part of this chapter, we discussed the direct effects of closed head injury on affective and behavioral functions interpretable as 'personality' factors. Most of these direct sequelae involve disruptions in functional unit I (hyper- or hypoarousal as interactive with affective behavior) and unit III ('frontal syndromes'). We turn now to a consideration of the ways in which changes in personality or behavior may reflect secondary or indirect effects of physical injury to the brain.

As we noted earlier, many of the personality changes reported by head injured patients or their relatives may be conceptualized as secondary to cognitive deficits which have a sweeping impact on typical patterns of behavior. For example, the patient who is unable to follow or contribute to conversations because of information processing inefficiency may eventually give up the attempt, earning the label of 'socially withdrawn'. Or he may attempt to regain the attention of others through socially unacceptable 'acting out'. In a related vein, *Levin and Grossman* [73] discuss the cognitively based 'failure to monitor or screen out irrelevant material' as a factor contributing to reports of psychiatric problems, particularly conceptual disorganization and emotional with-drawal, after severe head injury. Other changes in behavioral styles or patterns may be viewed as direct attempts to compensate for cognitive impairments. *Goldstein's* [74] well-known description of the 'cata-strophic reaction' to brain injury includes reports of patients who became orderly to the point of compulsion, apparently in an attempt to counteract the chaos induced by perceptual and cognitive changes. Any attempt to regain normal functioning, particularly in the face of *severe* or global alterations of memory, vision, language, or the ability to plan ahead, would necessitate drastic changes in premorbid behavior patterns and routines.

Just as cognitive deficits may lead to apparent changes in personal-ity and behavior, affective factors may color deficits which at first glance appear to be 'purely' cognitive. *Kline* [75] describes the interest-ing case of a young woman who suffered retrograde amnesia out of proportion to the severity of her head injury. The amnesia proved to be of hysterical origin, triggered by the similarity between the events preceding the head injury and emotionally traumatic events earlier in the patient's life. The retrograde amnesia was reversed by treatment with lithium carbonate. We treated a 13-year-old girl who sustained a severe head injury in an accident which killed several members of her family. This patient demonstrated inordinately severe memory deficits which failed to resolve over time or to respond to retraining efforts. We discovered that the patient believed that as her memory recovered, she would be able to recall the accident itself; this fear was exacerbated by hearing other family members describe the event in graphic detail. When the patient was convinced that she would never be able to remember the accident, there was marked improvement in her ante-rograde memory.

In addition to the specific behavioral or affective adaptations to cognitive sequelae described above, head-injured patients may be ex-pected to experience more general secondary reactions to physical, cognitive, and social changes. The field of rehabilitation psychology provides us with useful models of the affective changes which reliably follow a physical trauma resulting in disability. According to *Krueger* [76], there are five typical stages of reaction to physical disability:

(1) *Shock,* a state of emotional numbness in which the patient cannot comprehend the magnitude of the disabling event, may last from a few moments to several days.

(2) *Denial* normally persists for up to a week and acts as a necessary initial defense against the trauma.

(3) *Depression,* including feelings of grief, anger, lowered self esteem, and helplessness, signals the recognition of losses.

(4) *Reaction against independence* may appear as subversion of the gains achieved through rehabilitation. This stage is most commonly seen in adolescents or young adults for whom the struggles of autonomy and separation are relatively recent issues. It is particularly relevant to our discussion since head trauma predominantly affects this age group.

(5) *Adaptation* to the disability follows the effective development and use of coping strategies similar to those used in dealing with any major loss, such as the death of a loved one. These strategies may involve primarily affective means (e.g. denial), behavioral adaptations (e.g. immersion in activity, or acting-out), or cognitive mechanisms (information seeking, rationalization, projection, etc.).

Although these stages may provide a valid model for patients suffering from physical disabilities, it is questionable whether brain-injured patients experience the same progression toward adaptation or whether, in fact, they are capable of using many of the coping strategies cited by *Krueger*. During the period of confusion and post-traumatic amnesia, cognitive processes are, at best, disjointed and inconsistently applied. It is highly unlikely that patients in this stage are able to make consistent use of a coping strategy; in fact, most are not even fully aware of their disability. In later phases of recovery where there has developed some insight or recognition of the effects of the injury, a patient may attempt to use a coping strategy which has been successful in dealing with losses premorbidly. However, the old strategy may prove to be much less effective due to residual cognitive deficits. For example, the use of rationalization or the acquisition of information in order to gain intellectual control may be precluded by deficits in memory or reasoning. Likewise, a patient whose typical premorbid response to losses involved sharing feelings and reactions with others on a verbal level would be unable to cope in the usual way if he had suffered significant impairments in expressive language.

From the preceding discussion it is obvious that to assist the head-injured patient in dealing with losses incurred in the injury, the clinician must have a thorough understanding of the patient's cognitive status. This is necessary in order to aid the patient in substituting coping mechanisms which are feasible in light of residual cognitive deficits. Knowledge of neuropsychological status is also essential to avoid the misinterpretation of post-traumatic behavior patterns. We have seen, for example, patients with difficulty in initiating or maintaining behavior secondary to frontal lobe involvement labeled as 'passive-dependent' or 'resistant' to therapy efforts. Organically based deficits in self-evaluation may be erroneously interpreted as 'denial' in the psychoanalytic sense of the term. Such misunderstandings could lead to futile attempts at psychodynamically oriented psychotherapy which, in our experience, is inappropriate for all but the most cognitively intact head-injured patients. The level of abstraction necessary to benefit from this type of intervention is usually defective in these patients; in addition, they typically need a great deal more structure than is provided by psychodynamic therapies.

We have found that providing this structure in the form of brief verbal cues for adaptive coping strategies can be of excellent therapeutic value for patients with significant cognitive deficits. This procedure involves: (1) identifying premorbidly adaptive personality characteristics (e.g. assertiveness, persistence under stress) and current behavioral obstacles (e.g. passivity); (2) formulating a 'script' based on these characteristics, providing both a rationale and a means for coping (e.g. 'you've always been a tough survivor, now's the time to show it; stop being an innocent victim and come on like a Mack truck'), and (3) condensing from the script a cue which has meaning to the patient (e.g. 'Mack truck'). If the script is carefully developed and presented to the patient in a manner congruent with his current needs and cognitive limitations, the cue can eventually take on tremendous power in helping the patient through periods when he cannot develop effective strategies on his own. As treatment progresses, of course, the cues and their underlying scripts must be modified to meet new problems and goals.

Environmental Factors. In addition to the primary effects of the brain injury and the secondary emotional reactions to these effects, environmental factors can also contribute to affective and behavioral changes in patients with severe head injury. One particularly important environmental factor is the cumulative effect of weeks or months spent in a rehabilitation setting, where autonomy and control on the part of the patient are typically minimal or nonexistent. In the early stages of rehabilitation, there are obvious reasons for the loss of control: most patients are physically incapable of doing things for themselves or lack the rudimentary judgment necessary to make basic decisions. During recovery, the patient becomes gradually more competent but the typical rehabilitation unit continues to act for him, more out of convenience or efficiency than necessity. The patient may then persist in the 'sick role' with concomitant learned patterns of dependence on institutions and family members, even when the overt goal of the rehabilitation facility is that of helping him to achieve maximal independence. As expressed by *Keith* [77, p. 282]:

'American society has no really acceptable institutionalized model for disability. An individual is either well or sick. Hence the disabled person is forced into the sick role even if he may not want to assume it.'

An interesting parallel may be drawn to the phenomenon known as 'learned helplessness' [78], which has been proposed as one etiological factor in clinical depression. According to this model, a succession of *uncontrollable* stressors or traumatic events may induce characteristic affective and behavioral changes related to the cessation of attempts to control the environment. These changes include a decrease in response initiation, difficulty in learning response contingencies when the environment is actually controllable, and affective responses including anxiety and depression. It is all too easy to fit this model to a medical setting, where patients are necessarily subjected to painful and otherwise stressful events over which they have no control. In the case of the head injured patient, cognitive deficits may themselves interact with these environmental factors to exacerbate the helplessness and dependency. For example, a patient with organically based response initiation problems may have an even greater chance of learning that environmental events are not contingent on his behavior, which is emitted at a low rate to begin with. The effects of this learning would be to inhibit initiation even further, perpetuating a vicious cycle.

For these reasons, cognitive/behavioral therapy programs for the head injured should be designed so as to emphasize the contingency between patient behaviors and environmental events (both positive and negative) and to incorporate progressively greater requirements for initiation and autonomy. Consistent structuring of environmental contingencies can serve the dual purpose of restoring experiences of mastery and control to the patient, even as specific behaviors are being modified with the ultimate goal of reintegration to the social community [79, 80]. In addition, unlike the case of a circumscribed brain injury (such as stroke), the diffuse nature of head injury with its generalized effects on information processing dictates attention to *all* aspects of the environment as it interfaces with the patient's cognitive limitations. Therefore, environmental structuring is crucial to ensure that at each stage of recovery, the information processing demands of the setting are within the capabilities of the patient and that these demands are gradually increased to enhance cognitive recovery.

In considering the effects of the environment on affective and behavioral sequelae of head injury, the patient's premorbid personality and learning history are of critical importance in ways that are not fully understood. There is some evidence from the experimental literature on learned helplessness, for example, that certain individuals are more 'immune' to helplessness induced by uncontrollable stressors. The personality construct of locus of control appears to be important in this regard, in that people who already believe they are in control of environmental contingencies (i.e. those who have an internal locus of control) are more resistant to the development of learned helplessness [81]. Premorbid personality characteristics would not only contribute in this way but would, of course, color all of the affective and behavioral changes discussed thus far. For example, there is some evidence to suggest that premorbid 'instability' predisposes a head-injured patient to post-traumatic rage reactions [82]. Partly due to problems with the retrospective measurement of premorbid personality, there are few controlled studies in this area. The conventional wisdom that 'exaggeration of premorbid traits after injury is common' [50] is based mostly on anecdotal evidence.

In summary, effective treatment of the affective and behavioral sequelae of closed head injury involves attention to the origins of these dysfunctions and an integrated approach which considers the patient's cognitive status and both premorbid and post-traumatic coping styles. In both our inpatient and outpatient treatment programs, we have found the most successful approach to consist of environmental structuring with regard to information processing demands and the use of cueing (or 'scripting') and behavioral shaping procedures. Scripting serves the function of eliciting appropriate behaviors and coping strategies, while behavioral shaping reinforces the goal of autonomy and teaches the patient to function adaptively in a wider setting.

Effects on the Family

Any comprehensive attempt to provide treatment for the cognitive and behavioral sequelae of closed head injury must recognize the profound effects of such an injury on the patient's family. Particularly in the case of marital relationships, the incidence of discord, stress, and fragmentation in the family is very high [1, 17, 82, 83]. In general, family problems are more strongly associated with cognitive and personality changes than with residual physical disability [84].

A particularly valuable perspective from which to view the difficulties of the patient's family is provided by models of grief and bereavement. *Raphael* [85] defines bereavement as 'the reaction to the loss of a close relationship' (p. 33). We would argue that bereavement *must* occur in some form in the relatives and close companions of a patient whose cognitive and/or personality changes are such as to alter the nature of the interpersonal relationship. Even changes that appear minor to an outsider, such as 'subtle' alterations in drive, social inhibition, or sensitivity to others, may translate to significant losses in a close relationship such as marriage.

Bereavement following the death of a loved one occurs in several stages [85]: After a period of shock and disbelief, the bereaved feels intense pain caused by the absence of the loved one. Anger, longing, sadness, and helplessness are experienced. However, over time the *continued* absence of the lost person (as well as participation in rituals for 'disposing of the body') forces the gradual recognition that the loss is permanent. The finality of the loss is progressively reinforced until some level of acceptance occurs. Now the bereaved is ready to review the many bonds that built the relationship, and relinquish them: 'As mourning progresses, the bonds are undone, the emotions freed for reinvestment in life once more' (p. 46).

The pattern of response to the loss of a close relationship after head injury is entirely different. The normal grieving process is necessarily disorganized, leading to what *Rosenthal and Muir* [86] called 'mobile mourning'. In the first place, families are seldom certain as to what aspects of the relationship must be mourned, since the permanent losses are difficult to predict. Secondly, the eventual acceptance of the loss is complicated by the physical presence of the 'lost' person [84]. Not only does the presence of the loved one prevent the realization of the finality of loss; but his presence in 'altered form' provides a continual painful reminder of the ways in which a close relationship was changed.

Finally, during the mourning phase in which affective bonds are freed for reinvestment elsewhere, the bereaved person is faced with the nearly impossible task of maintaining a relationship with the altered person while mourning the relationship they had previously enjoyed.

Different families, of course, find different ways of dealing with this very difficult situation. A common reaction is denial, either of the loss itself or of its magnitude or significance [87]. Some family members must separate themselves physically from the patient in order to complete the mourning process; in our experience, this occurs more frequently with spouses than with parents or children. Others are able to remain physical contact with the patient, even to the point of providing care, while managing to withdraw *all* emotional investment from the relationship. Still others are eventually able to mourn the losses but keep the bonds that are appropriate to building a new relationship with the altered person.

In marital relationships which do remain intact after severe head trauma, changes in sexual functioning frequently provide yet another source of stress. Head injury has the potential for affecting the sexual relationship at many levels: At the *neuronal* level there can be changes in hormone function or brain lesions which directly cause hyper- or hypoarousal; *physical* changes may affect mobility and body image; *sensory* deficits such as decreased tactile sensation, anosmia, or loss of visual imagery may affect arousal; and relevant *cognitive and behavioral* changes may include distractibility, disinhibition, and egocentricity. In addition, secondary emotional responses such as fear of impotence, feelings of unattractiveness, and loss of self-confidence can undermine sexual functioning. Changes in the sexual relationship can obviously generate a significant degree of conflict for the patient's spouse. We have known wives of head-injured patients who felt that the sexual relationship had changed so much that they were being 'unfaithful' to their husbands.

Treatment Issues. Intervention for family difficulties is approached in different ways at different institutions. However, on many rehabilitation units it is standard procedure for the family to be interviewed (prior to admission, if possible) by a family counselor or social services representative. The purposes of this interview are: (1) to gather information about the patient's premorbid personality, social status, and

role within the family unit; (2) to ascertain the family's level of understanding and acceptance of the injury and its sequelae, and to assess
their current methods of coping, and (3) to initiate a therapeutic relationship with the family, for the purpose of offering information and
emotional support.

Most state-of-the-art head injury rehabilitation programs offer
ongoing education and support groups for family members [86]. These
serve an important function in reducing the stress associated with the
uncertainties of the acute rehabilitation phase, particularly if counseling in specific stress management techniques is provided. However, the
clinician should keep in mind that not all techniques are appropriate
for all families participating in a group. For example, relaxation training using visual imagery would be contraindicated for a family member
who is disturbed by recurring images related to the trauma.

Our experience with these counseling groups, and with other forms
of family intervention in the inpatient setting, is that a subset of the
family members who choose *not* to take advantage of these services are
the ones who turn out to be most at risk. These individuals often appear
unusually cheerful, failing to express any 'negative' affect at all. If not
handled properly, they will attempt to avoid all contact with rehabilitation professionals. Since these people are clearly not ready to *receive*
information, we maintain contact with them by asking them to *give*
information to us. Typically, we would initiate contact by explaining
that there are often valid reasons to expect discrepancies between staff
perceptions and family perceptions of the patient's condition and progress. Families can then be asked to keep track of certain aspects of the
patient's behavior with the goal of meeting regularly with a staff member to 'compare notes'. We have found that letting these families know
that we need their information, rather than trying to force our information on them, is a valuable way of maintaining contact long enough to
build the rapport needed for strategic intervention when the family is
ready.

Late-Stage Rehabilitation: Social and Vocational Re-Entry

For most patients with severe closed head injury, the rehabilitation
process is far from complete at the point of discharge from an inpatient
facility. Even those who have received state-of-the-art medical, physi-

cal, and psychological interventions face a bleak prognosis for returning to a level of function approaching their premorbid status [88]. Head-injured individuals may function at a deceptively high level in the hospital setting, yet upon discharge will experience social isolation and withdrawal, disruption in family relationships, and extreme difficulty in coping with the demands of full-time occupation. *Malkmus* [47, p. 1959] expressed the problem well:

> 'Although cognitive function . . . is improved at this phase of recovery, if environmental structure and predictability are altered, performance will be altered as well. The individual's inability to integrate his increased cognitive, physical, and emotional capacities into the real world will become apparent.'

A great many head-injured individuals with residual deficits in information processing are simply incapable of coping with the speed, pressure, stress, and complexity of the 'real world' without specialized late-stage intervention. In recent years, a number of programs have been developed specifically to assist the re-entry of these patients into satisfactory social and vocational roles. We will discuss briefly the major components of these programs using our own, project re-entry, as an illustration. Project Re-Entry is a full-time, intensive outpatient program originally modeled on the head trauma program at the New York University Institute of Rehabilitation Medicine [89]. It is also quite similar in overall structure and philosophy to the pioneering project described by *Rosenbaum* et al. [90].

Program Components

Project Re-Entry consists of the following treatment modalities, attended daily. *Cognitive retraining* provides practice and compensatory strategies to overcome or adapt to residual deficits in memory, communication, reasoning, and visual perception. *Stress management,* in the form of biofeedback and relaxation training, is included to counteract the head injured patient's disproportionate response to stress. *Psychotherapeutic intervention* in a group format focuses on interpersonal skills and coping strategies for dealing with the effects of the injury. It involves more behavioral intervention and individualized 'scripting' than psychodynamic therapy, for the reasons outlined earlier. *Group exercises* with both structured and unstructured formats provide an opportunity for practicing cognitive and interpersonal skills and receiving feedback from peers. *Leisure time and community resources* are addressed to help provide the patient with new or alterate sources of gratification and to enhance socialization. *Vocational training* includes an assessment of skills, interests, and aptitudes, training in basic skills such as interviewing, and attention to compensatory strategies for cognitive and interpersonal limitations in the work setting. Upon 'graduation' from the therapy phase of Project Re-Entry, patients are placed in a therapeutic job trial within the hospital which is closely monitored by trained vocational counselors. Eventually, the patient is assisted in finding a permanent job placement, at the competitive level in most cases.

Process Variables Related to Success

Our experience with the development and implementation of Project Re-Entry has allowed us to identify the following process variables as crucial to the success of this and similar programs. *Group treatment* is essential at this stage of rehabilitation for the full development of insight into the effects of the injury [79] and for the acquisition of adaptive coping strategies. In addition, a group format allows intensive work on interpersonal and social skills which would be impossible with one-on-one treatment.

Gradual decrease in structure with an increase in stress is built into every aspect of the program. Patients are expected to assume progressively more autonomy and handle more pressure until task conditions approximate those of complex social and vocational activities. *Integration of program components,* which is essential, is achieved in several ways. First, for each patient, key treatment issues are targeted and addressed in a consistent way across all treatment modalities. Second, in the later stages of treatment the content of the therapies is deliberately 'blended'. In the advanced phase of cognitive retraining, for example, patients perform exercises which combine cognitive and interpersonal aspects of communication, and work on group projects which simulate vocational activities. *Family involvement* is achieved by meeting with significant family members every 6 weeks, to update them on the patient's progress and to observe family dynamics which will affect the therapeutic process. *Long-term vocational follow-up* has proved to be crucial to the ultimate success of the program. Even after patients are placed in competitive employment, intermittent contact with them and their employers is necessary to maintain gains achieved in rehabilitation and to forestall new problems.

Conclusion: Implications for the Rehabilitation Team

The successful rehabilitation of the severely head-injured adult is a complex problem, the solution of which is still in its infancy. The design and implementation of effective programs for this population depends on a thorough understanding of the pathophysiology of head injury and its typical cognitive and behavioral correlates. Head trauma frequently affects the neural substrate for nonspecific functions such as arousal and attention in the 'cognitive' sphere and overall self-monitoring in the 'behavioral' sphere. Because disturbances in these nonspecific functions impact nearly all aspects of adaptive behavior, interventions for head injury must be both multifaceted and interdisciplinary at every stage of recovery.

We would like to conclude with some comments on this concept of *interdisciplinary* rehabilitation. As we have discussed, our experience indicates that successful treatment for this population includes: environmental structuring which is carefully suited to the patient's information processing capabilities; scripting to elicit appropriate behaviors and coping strategies; and behavioral shaping. This treatment approach requires a highly consistent attitude from all staff members who come into contact with a patient. If the rehabilitation team consists of professionals from diverse fields each 'doing their own thing' with a minimum of communication among them, the treatment effort is doomed to failure. We would consider such a team to be *multidisciplinary* rather than interdisciplinary. In an interdisciplinary approach, each team member's primary task is to reinforce the agreed-upon environmental strategies targeted for each patient. Thus, regardless of his or her professional speciality, each team member is first and foremost a behavioral manager, and secondly a professional responsible for a particular aspect of the patient's care and training. The interdisciplinary approach [91] requires a great deal of overlap among professional specialities, and a willingness to 'make a deliberate attempt to achieve a blurring of roles, which provides a "consistency of expectation".' This concept is a familiar one in many mental health settings [92], but is still foreign to rehabilitation units where boundaries have been carefully staked and territories jealously guarded. It is our hope that the continued success of the interdisciplinary team will make it the standard approach to the treatment of severe head injury.

References

1 Thomsen, I.V.: The patient with severe head injury and his family. Scand. J. Rehabil. Med. *6:* 180–183 (1974).

2 Brooks, N.: Head injury and the family; in Brooks, Closed head injury: psychological, social, and family consequences (Oxford Press, Oxford 1984).

3 Jennett, B.; Teasdale, G.: Management of head injuries (Davies, Philadelphia 1981).

4 Levin, H.S.; Benton, A.L.; Grossman, R.G.: Neurobehavioral consequences of closed head injury (Oxford Press, New York 1982).

5 Luria, A.R.: The working brain (Basic Books, New York 1973).

6 Ommaya, A.K.; Gennarelli, T.I.: Cerebral concussion and traumatic unconsciousness. Correlations of experimental and clinical observations on blunt head injuries. Brain *97:* 633–654 (1974).

7 Plum, F.; Posner, J.: The diagnosis of stupor and coma (Davis, Philadelphia 1980).

8 Adams, J.H.; Mitchell, D.E.; Graham, D.I.; Doyle, D.: Diffuse brain damage of immediate impact type. Brain *100:* 489–502 (1977).

9 Mitchell, D.E.; Adams, J.H.: Primary focal impact damage to the brain-stem in blunt head injuries. Does it exist? Lancet *ii:* 215–218 (1973).

10 Lindenberg, R.; Freytag, E.: Brainstem lesions characteristic of traumatic hypertension of the head. Archs Path. *90:* 509–515 (1970).

11 Teasdale, G.; Mendelow, D.: Pathophysiology of head injuries; in Brooks, Closed head injury: psychological, social, and family consequences (Oxford Press, Oxford 1984).

12 Conkey, R.C.: Psychological changes associated with head injuries. Archs Psychol. *33:* 1–62 (1938).

13 Van Zomeren, A.H.; Brouwer, W.H.; Deelman, B.G.: Attentional deficits: The riddles of selectivity, speed, and alertness; in Brooks, Closed head injury: psychological, social, and family consequences (Oxford Press, Oxford 1984).

14 Gronwall, D.; Sampson, H.: The psychological effects of concussion (Auckland University Press, Auckland 1974).

15 Gronwall, D.; Wrightson, P.: Delayed recovery of intellectual function after minor head injury. Lancet *ii:* 605–609 (1974).

16 Minderhound, J.M.; Van Woerkom, T.C.A.M.; Van Weerden, T.W.: On the nature of brainstem disorders in severe head-injured patients. II. A study on caloric vestibular reactions and neurotransmitter treatment. Acta neurochir. *34:* 32–35 (1976).

17 Ommaya, A.K.: Reintegrative action of the nervous system after trauma; in Popp, Neural trauma (Raven Press, New York 1979).

18 Butters, N.: Amnesic disorders; in Heilman, Valenstein, Clinical neuropsychology (Oxford Press, New York 1979).

19 Brooks, N.: Cognitive deficits after head injury; in Brooks, Closed head injury: psychological, social, and family consequences (Oxford Press, Oxford 1984) (b).

20 Buschke, H.; Fuld, P.A.: Evaluating storage, retention and retrieval in disordered memory and learning. Neurology, Minneap. *24:* 1019–1025 (1974).

21 Hannay, H.J.; Levin, H.S.; Grossman, R.G.: Impaired recognition memory after head injury. Cortex *15:* 269–283 (1979).

22   Schacter, S.: The interaction of cognitive and physiological determinants of emotional state; in Berkowitz, Advances in experimental social psychology, vol. I (Academic Press, New York 1970).

23   Valenstein, E.; Heilman, K.M.: Emotional disorders resulting from lesions of the central nervous system; in Heilman, Valenstein, Clinical neuropsychology (Oxford Press, New York 1979).

24   Damasio, A.; Van Hoesen, G.W.: Emotional disturbances associated with focal lesions of the limbic frontal lobe; in Heilman, Satz, Neuropsychology of human emotion (Guilford, New York 1983).

25   Lishman, W.A.: The psychiatric sequelae of head injury. A review. Psychol. Med. 3: 304–318 (1973).

26   Adams, J.H.; Scott, G.; Parker, L.S.; Graham, D.I.; Doyle, D.: The contusion index. A quantitative approach to cerebral contusion in head injury. Neuropathol. appl. Neurobiol. 6: 319–324 (1980).

27   Russell, W.R.: Injury to cranial nerves and optic chiasm; in Brock, Injuries of the brain and spinal cord and their coverings, 4th ed. (Springer, New York 1960).

28   Crompton, M.R.: Visual lesion in closed head injury. Brain 93: 785–792 (1970).

29   Ruesch, J.: Dark adaptation, negative after images, tachistoscopic examinations and reaction time in head injuries. J. Neurosurg. 1: 243–251 (1944).

30   Hannay, H.J.; Levin, H.S.; Kay, M.: Tachistoscopic visual perception after closed head injury. J. clin. Neuropsychol. 4: 117–129 (1982).

31   Levin, H.S.; Peters, B.H.: Neuropsychological testing following closed head injuries. Prosopagnosia without visual field defect. Dis. nerv. Syst. 37: 68–71 (1976).

32   Dikmen, S.; Reitan, R.M.; Temkin, N.R.: Neuropsychological recovery in head injury. Archs Neurol. 40: 333–338 (1983).

33   Heilman, K.M.; Scholes, R.; Watson, R.T.: Auditory affective agnosia: Disturbed comprehension of affective speech. J. Neurol. Neurosurg. Psychiat. 38: 69–72 (1975).

34   Damasio, A.: The frontal lobes; in Heilman, Valenstein, Clinical neuropsychology (Oxford Press, New York 1979).

35   Stuss, D.T.; Benson, D.F.: Neuropsychological studies of the frontal lobes. Psychol. Bull. 95: 3–28 (1984).

36   Lezak, M.D.: Neuropsychological assessment; 2nd ed. (Oxford Press, New York 1983).

37   Mandleberg, I.A.; Brooks, D.N.: Cognitive recovery after severe head injury. I. Serial testing on the Wechsler Adult Intelligence Scale. J. Neurol. Neurosurg. Psychiat. 38: 1121–1126 (1975).

38   Blumer, D.; Benson, D.F.: Personality changes with frontal and temporal lobe lesions; in Benson, Blumer, Psychiatric aspects of neurological disease (Grune & Stratton, New York 1975).

39   Bricolo, A.; Turazzi, S.; Feriotti, G.: Prolonged posttraumatic unconsciousness: Therapeutic assets and liabilities. J. Neurosurg. 52: 625–634 (1980).

40   Champlin, L.: Beyond simple survival. Today's Nursing Home 3: 20 (1982).

41   Luria, A.R.; Naydin, V.L.; Tsvetkova, L.S.; Vinarskaya, E.N.: Restoration of higher cortical function following local brain damage; in Vinkin, Bruyn, Handbook of clinical neurology, vol. III (North-Holland, Amsterdam 1969).

42 Weber, P.L.: Sensorimotor therapy. Its effect on electroencephalograms of acute comatose patients. Archs phys. Med. Rehabil. *65:* 457–462 (1984).

43 Boyle, M.E.; Greer, R.D.: Operant procedures and the comatose patient. J. appl. Behav. Anal. *16:* 3–12 (1983).

44 Leon, M.; Snyder, M.: Care of the long-term comatose patient. A pilot study. J. Neurosurg. Nurs. *12:* 134–137 (1980).

45 Tobis, J.S.; Puri, K.B.; Sheridan, J.: Rehabilitation of the severely brain-injured patient. Scand. J. rehab. Med. *14:* 83–88 (1982).

46 Fauman, M.A.: Treatment of the agitated patient with an organic brain disorder. J. Am: med. Ass. *240:* 380–382 (1978).

47 Malkmus, D.: Integrating cognitive strategies into the physical therapy setting. Phys. Ther. *63:* 1952–1959 (1983).

48 Olson, D.A.; Henig, E.: A manual of behavior management strategies for traumatically brain-injured adults (Rehabilitation Institute of Chicago, Chicago 1983).

49 Feeney, D.M.; Gonzalez, A.; Law, W.A.: Amphetamine, haloperidol, and experience interact to affect rate of recovery after motor cortex injury. Science *217:* 855–857 (1982).

50 Bond, M. The psychiatry of closed head injury; in Brooks, Closed head injury: psychological, social, and family consequences (Oxford Press, Oxford 1984).

51 Gans, J.S.: Hate in the rehabilitation setting. Archs phys. Med. Rehabil. *64:* 176–179 (1983).

52 Patten, B.M.: The ancient art of memory: usefulness in treatment. Archs Neurol. *26:* 25–31 (1972).

53 Jones, M.K.: Imagery as a mnemonic aid after left temporal lobectomy. Contrast between material-specific and generalized memory disorders. Neuropsychologia *12:* 21–30 (1974).

54 Lewinsohn, P.; Danaher, B.; Kikel, S.: Visual imagery as a mnemonic aid for brain injured persons. J. consult. clin. Psychol. *45:* 717–723 (1977).

55 Gasparrini, B.; Satz, P.: A treatment for memory problems in left hemisphere CVA patients. J. clin. Neuropsychol. *1:* 137–150 (1979).

56 Podbros, L.Z.; Noble, P.B.: Elaboration strategies. Their effect on memory retention in two amnesic patients. Congr. Physical Medicine and Rehabilitation, Houston 1982.

57 Crovitz, H.: Memory retraining in brain-damaged patients. The airplane list. Cortex *15:* 131–134 (1979).

58 Gianutsos, R.; Gianutsos, J.: Rehabilitating the verbal recall of brain-injured patients by mnemonic training. An experimental demonstration using single-case methodology. J. clin. Neuropsychol. *1:* 117–135 (1979).

59 Gianutsos, R.: Training the short- and long-term verbal recall of a post-encephalitic amnesic. J. clin. Neuropsychol. *3:* 143–153 (1981).

60 Kovner, R.; Mattis, S.; Goldmeier, E.: A technique for promoting robust free recall in chronic organic amnesia. J. clin. Neuropsychol. *5:* 65–71 (1983).

61 Luria, A.R.: Restoration of function after brain injury (MacMillan, New York 1963).

62 Albert, M.L.; Sparks, R.W.; Helm, N.A.: Melodic intonation therapy for aphasia. Archs Neurol. *29:* 130–131 (1973).

63 Gardner, H.; Zurif, E.B.; Berry, T.; Baker, E.: Visual communication in aphasia. Neuropsychologia *14:* 275–292 (1976).

64 Diller, L; Weinberg, J.: Hemi-inattention in rehabilitation. The evolution of a rational remediation program; in Weinstein, Friedland, Advances in neurology, vol. 18 (Raven Press, New York 1977).

65 Weinberg, J.; Diller, L.; Gordon, W.A.; Gerstman, L.J.; Lieberman, A.; Lakin, P.; Hodges, G.; Ezrachi, O.: Visual scanning training effect on reading-related tasks in acquired brain damage. Archs phys. Med. Rehabil. *58:* 479–486 (1977).

66 Weinberg, J.; Piasetsky, E.; Diller, L.; Gordon, W.: Treating perceptual organization deficits in nonneglecting RBD stroke patients. J. clin. Neuropsychol. *4:* 59–75 (1982).

67 Diller, L.; Ben-Yishay, Y.; Gerstman, L.J.; Goodkin, R.; Gordon, W.; Weinberg, J.: Studies in cognitive and rehabilitation in hemiplegia (New York University Institute of Rehabilitation Medicine, New York 1974).

68 Diller, L.; Gordon, W.: Interventions for cognitive deficits in brain-injured adults. J. consult. clin. Psychol. *49:* 822–834 (1981).

69 Heaton, R.K.; Pendleton, M.G.: Use of neuropsychological tests to predict adult patients' everyday functioning. J. consult. clin. Psychol. *49:* 807–821 (1981).

70 Jennett, B.; Snoek, J.; Bond, M.R.; Brooks, D.N.: Disability after severe head injury. Observations in the use of the Glasgow Outcome Scale. J. Neurol. Neurosurg. Psychiat. *44:* 285–293 (1981).

71 Brooks, N.; McKinlay, W.: Personality and behavioral change after severe blunt head injury. A relative's view. J. Neurol. Neurosurg. Psychiat. *46:* 336–344 (1983).

72 Fordyce, D.J.; Roueche, J.R.; Prigatano, G.P.: Enhanced emotional reactions in chronic head trauma patients. J. Neurol. Neurosurg. Psychiat. *46:* 620–624 (1983).

73 Levin, H.S.; Grossman, R.G.: Behavioral sequelae of closed head injury. A quantitative study. Archs Neurol. *35:* 720–727 (1978).

74 Goldstein, K.: The effect of brain damage on the personality. Psychiatry *15:* 245–260 (1952).

75 Kline, N.A.: Reversal of post-traumatic amnesia with lithium. Psychosomatics *20:* 363–364 (1979).

76 Krueger, D.W.: Psychological rehabilitation of physical trauma and disability; in Krueger, Rehabilitation psychology (Aspen, Rockville 1984).

77 Keith, R.A.: The need for a new model in rehabilitation. J. chron. Dis. *21:* 281–286 (1978).

78 Seligman, M.E.P.: Helplessness: on depression, development, and death (Freeman, San Francisco 1975).

79 Newcombe, F.: The psychological consequences of closed head injury. Assessment and rehabilitation. Injury *14:* 11–136 (1973).

80 Wood, R.L.: Behaviour disorder following severe brain injury: Their presentation and psychological management; in Brooks, Closed head injury: psychological, social, and family consequences (Oxford Press, Oxford 1984).

81 Hiroto, D.S.: Locus of control and learned helplessness. J. exp. Psychol. *102:* 187–193 (1974).

82 Panting, A.; Merry, P.: The long-term rehabilitation of severe head injuries with particular references to the need for social and medical support for the patient's family. Rehabilitation *38:* 33–37 (1972).

83   Thomsen, I.V.: Late outcome of very severe blunt head trauma. A 10–15 year
      second follow-up. J. Neurol. Neurosurg. Psychiat. *47:* 260–268 (1984).
84   Bond, M.: Effects on the family system; in Rosenthal, Griffith, Bond, Miller,
      Rehabilitation of the head injured adult (Davis, Philadelphia 1983).
85   Raphael, B.: The anatomy of bereavement (Basic Books, New York 1982).
86   Rosenthal, M.; Muir, C.A.: Methods of family intervention; in Rosenthal, Griffith,
      Bond, Miller, Rehabilitation of the head injured adult. (Davis, Philadelphia 1983).
87   Romano, M.D.: Family response to traumatic head injury. Scand. J. Rehabil. Med.
      6: 1–4 (1974).
88   Oddy, M.: Head injury and social adjustment; in Brooks, Closed head injury:
      psychological, social, and family consequences (Oxford Press, Oxford 1984).
89   Ben-Yishay, Y.: Working approaches to remediation of cognitive deficits in brain
      damaged persons (New York University Institute of Rehabilitation Medicine, New
      York 1980).
90   Rosenbaum, M.; Lipsitz, N.; Abraham, J.; Najenson, T.: A description of an
      intensive treatment project for the rehabilitation of severely brain-injured soldiers.
      Scand. J. Rehabil. Med. *10:* 1–6 (1978).
91   Goodman-Smith, A.; Turnbull, J.: A behavioural approach to the rehabilitation of
      severely brain-injured adults. Physiotherapy *69:* 393–396 (1983).
92   Almond, R.: The healing community: dynamics of the therapeutic milieu (Jason
      Aronson, New York 1974).

Mary Ellen Hayden, PhD, Director of Neuropsychology, Medical Center Del Oro,
Houston, TX 77002 (USA)

Subject Index